Honey in Modern Wound Management

Other titles available from Wounds UK include:

Skin Care in Wound Management: Assessment, prevention and treatment
edited by Richard White

A Pocket Guide to Clinical Decision-making in Wound Management
edited by Sue Bale and David Gray

Paediatric Skin and Wound Care
edited by Richard White and Jacqueline Denyer

Trauma and Pain in Wound Care, volume I
edited by Richard White and Keith Harding

Leg Ulcers and Problems of the Lower Limb: An holistic approach
edited by Ellie Lindsay and Richard White

Advances in Wound Care, volume I
edited by Richard White

Trauma and Pain in Wound Care, volume II
edited by Richard White and Keith Harding

VAC Therapy: An introduction and practical guide
edited by David Gray, Fiona Russell and John Timmons

Honey in Modern Wound Management

edited by
Rose Cooper, Peter Molan and Richard White

Wounds UK
—— Publishing ——

HealthComm UK Limited, trading as Wounds UK Limited, Suite 3.1,
36 Upperkirkgate, Aberdeen AB10 1BA

British Library Cataloguing-in-Publication Data
A catalogue record is available for this book

ISBN-10 0-9555758-5-0
ISBN-13 978-0-9555758-5-3

Printed in Malta by Gutenberg Press Limited, Tarxien, Malta

CONTENTS

CONTRIBUTORS

Julie Betts is Nurse Practitioner in Wound Care, Waikato District Health Board, Hamilton, New Zealand

Shona Blair is Postdoctoral Research Fellow, School of Molecular and Microbial Biosciences, University of Sydney, Australia

Gisela Blaser is Wound Care Specialist, Study Nurse. Woundviewer Database, Children's Hospital Medical Center, University of Bonn, Germany

Laura Bolton is Adjunct Associate Professor, Department of Surgery (Bioengineering), University of Medicine and Dentistry of New Jersey and Chief Scientific Advisor, Derma Sciences Inc, Princeton, and President, Scientific Consulting with Integrity (SCI) LLC, New Jersey, USA

Rose Cooper is Professor of Microbiology, Cardiff School of Health Sciences, University of Wales Institute Cardiff (UWIC), Cardiff, Wales

Stuart Enoch is Speciality Registrar in Burns and Plastic Surgery, Department of Burns and Plastic Surgery, University Hospital of South Manchester and Manchester University Children's Hospitals, Manchester

Robert Frykberg is Chief Podiatrist, Carl T Hayden Veterans Affairs Medical Centre and Clinics, Phoenix, Arizona, USA

Georgina Gethin is Lecturer, Research Centre, Faculty of Nursing and Midwifery, Royal College of Surgeons in Ireland (RCSI), Dublin, Ireland

Chris Hill is General Manager, Manuka Medical Ltd, Mansfield, Nottingham

David Johnson is Director of Nephrology, Chair of Medicine, Professor of Medicine (University of Queensland), Professor of Population Health (University of Queensland), Princess Alexandra Hospital, Woolloongabba, Brisbane, Australia

Caroline McIntosh is Senior Lecturer, Department of Podiatry, National University of Ireland, Galway, Ireland

Rhianna Miles is Advanced Trainee in Renal Medicine, Department of Nephrology, Princess Alexandra Hospital, Woolloongabba, Brisbane, Australia

Peter Molan is Professor in Biological Sciences and Director of the Honey Research Unit, University of Waikato, Hamilton, New Zealand

Val Robson is Clinical Nurse Specialist, Leg Ulcer Care, Aintree Hospitals NHS Trust, Liverpool

Kai Santos is Wound Care Specialist, Study Coordinator. Woundviewer Database, Children's Hospital Medical Center, University of Bonn, Germany

Arne Simon is Consultant in Paediatric, Haematology and Oncology, Paediatric Infectious Diseases, Children's Hospital Medical Center, University of Bonn, Germany; Member of the Commission for Hospital Hygiene and Prevention of Infection, Robert Kock Institute, Berlin and Member of the Directorate of the German Society of Hospital Hygiene (DGKH)

Mutya Subrahmanyam is Professor and Head, Department of Surgery, Bharati Vidyapeeth University Medical College and Hospital, Sangli, Maharashtra, India

Amanda Tonks is Lecturer, Department of Microbiology, School of Medicine, Cardiff University, Cardiff

PREFACE

Since the publication by Wounds UK of the first book on honey as a modern wound management product, the use of medical grade honey in treating a diverse range of wounds has accelerated dramatically. As a consequence, many patients have experienced the multiple benefits of its unique healing properties. In an age where technological advancement is all around us, the fact that a pure, natural product that was originally used thousands of years ago is now widely selected for extensive, modern clinical use is testament to its exceptional properties.

This increased use has led to a significant rise in the amount of clinical evidence and has generated interest in an expanding number of countries. The range of licensed products available has expanded from sterile honey in tubes to a broader range of devices, with more advanced dressings now available. As a result, medical grade honey is often the first choice of dressing for many healthcare professionals, fulfilling not only their clinical demands, but also satisfying cost-effective requirements.

This book not only provides reviews of clinical data, but also technical information and expert opinion. The authors are drawn from four continents and reflect the varying therapeutic applications of honey, making it an ideal reference book for all healthcare professionals. This wealth of knowledge will allow anyone unfamiliar with honey, or those still unsure of its benefits, to evaluate the evidence and form valuable insights into its potential.

Advancis Medical would like to recognise the contribution from all the authors and the clinical professionals who have participated in compiling this book.

Mark Allatt
Sales and Marketing Director
Advancis Medical
October, 2008

FOREWORD

One late Friday afternoon some 25 years ago, as I trudged up a long steep corridor in the hospital, a senior clinician fell into step with me and began a conversation about my research studies in wound healing. At that time I was a research novice trying to study tissue microcirculation. Unable to edit my thoughts at short notice, I began to mumble about some of my observations. 'Any thoughts on how we can treat these wounds?' he asked and without waiting for a response said, 'Honey works you know — we used it years ago when I was training'.

I was to recall his words a decade later after initiating the Cochrane Wounds Groups (CWG) which heralded the availability of high quality data related to clinical effectiveness in wound healing. The CWG has produced Level 1 evidence based on randomised controlled studies relating some well used interventions. We understand the positive implications of such reports and that they apply to the population who may be fitted into a distribution curve. But, what are we to do about patients who fall outside this curve? Can we identify such wounds and how are we to treat their wounds with confidence?

As many authors have described, honey has been used to treat wounds for many centuries. The editors of this book have covered a spectrum of analytical and other studies of different types of honey in their research. This book gives the reader the latest thoughts on the composition and the value of using honeys to treat chronic wounds of different aetiologies. The reader should welcome the opportunity to read and understand this seminal text led by top scientists in their field.

The role of honey in wound management is a question that I often encounter. A book such as this will be an invaluable resource to all: to those who should know the answers but do not, as well as those who would like to know and are eager to learn.

Dr Raj Mani
Head of Clinical Measurements and Senior Lecturer
Director of Vascular Laboratory, Division of Diagnostics and Therapies
Southampton University Hospitals Trust, Southampton

INTRODUCTION

Over the last decades, advances in knowledge of wound healing have grown rapidly. More and more information is published every day on exciting molecules targeting diverse components and cells involved in regaining skin integrity. Healthcare professionals face new challenges, such as inflammation and infection control without causing further damage to the fragile structure developing inside a healing wound. Furthermore, as technology advances, products become increasingly expensive and, therefore, impractical in many parts of the world where resources are scarce.

Honey is probably the oldest documented remedy used for wound care that we are aware of, as it was used by the Egyptians and recorded in the Ebers papyrus. Its use has not only survived until today, but we are finding that it has more and more properties. The editors and contributors to this book have made an excellent compendium of the new evidence and research into the use of honey in wound care, with the debate revolving around new discoveries in the mechanism of action of honey, and the clinical evidence of its applicability and use in different types of wounds.

The text provides the reader with enough information to understand what honey can and cannot do and, more importantly, becomes the base upon which many new questions arise, opening a window for research especially related to its use in underserved countries.

This book has been long awaited and the reader will be surprised by the sheer amount of new information inside these pages: knowledge that will be of use to the clinician, the researcher, the biologist and anyone with an interest in this still mysterious compound.

José Contreras-Ruiz
Interdisciplinary Wound and Ostomy Care Centre
'Dr. Manuel Gea González' General Hospital
Mexico City, Mexico
October, 2008

Editor's note

Since going to press two systematic reviews of the clinical efficacy of honey have been published:

Bardy J, Slevin NJ, Mais KL, Molassiotis A (2008) A systematic review of honey uses and its potential value within oncology care. *J Clinical Nursing* 17: 2604–23

Jull AB, Rodgers A, Walker N (2008) Honey as a topical treatment for wounds. *Cochrane Database of Systematic Reviews* 2008, Issue 4. Art. No: CD005083

But for the timing of their availability, these papers may well have been included in several of the chapters within this book,

Rose Cooper
14 October, 2008

CHAPTER 1

AN HISTORICAL INTRODUCTION TO THE MEDICINAL USE OF HONEY

Shona Blair

Honey has been used as a medicine throughout the history of the human race, and one of the most common and persistent therapeutic uses of honey has been as a wound dressing. Without doubt, a considerable component in the endurance of honey as a medicine is its significant antibacterial activity, which is discussed in *Chapters* 3 and 4.

A brief history of the medicinal use of honey

Some of the earliest rock art, which has been found in such diverse places as Africa, Australia, India, Bhutan, Spain and Sri Lanka, depicts the collection of honey. The configuration of these pictures, and the fact that they were often preserved rather than painted over, indicates that honey was held in high regard and deemed to possess considerable power (Crane, 1986; Crane, 1999; Crane, 2001). In many cultures there was often an overlap between magic, religion and medicine. Honey and/or bees were held as sacred in numerous religions for at least some stage throughout their history, if not constantly. These include Aryan Veda (later Hinduism), Buddhism, Christianity, Confucianism, Ancient Egyptian cults, Greek cults, Islam, Ancient Israeli (later Judaism), Persian Sects, prehistoric religions, Roman cults, Shinto, Sikhism and Taoism. In addition, many sacred texts, such as the Bible, Qur'an and Torah, specifically mention the medicinal use of honey (Beck, 1938; Crane, 1999; Lev, 2003).

Humans initially hunted for honey, and numerous peoples robbed wild hives to obtain it, usually destroying the colony in the process. The Ancient Egyptians were among the first beekeepers, rather than honey hunters. Around 3500 BC Upper and Lower Egypt were united under one ruler and the hieroglyph of a bee first appeared, denoting the king of Lower Egypt (Ransome, 1937). It is possible that beekeeping started as early as 5000 BC and it was well established by the First Dynasty, around 3100 BC (Crane, 1999). Apiculture as a profession was illustrated in temples and the pictures include the Egyptian beekeepers using smoke to pacify the bees while robbing their hives of honey (Darby *et al*, 1977). The Egyptians moved hives up and down the Nile to follow the nectar flow from different flowering plants as the seasons changed (Ransome, 1937).

Records found in papyrus documents tell that honey was used extensively in Egyptian medicine. The Edwin Smith Surgical Papyrus dates back to around 1700 BC, but is thought to contain knowledge from a much earlier era, possibly 3000–2500 BC. This text appears to be a surgical textbook, describing 48 cases and how to examine, diagnose, and treat them. Honey is a common ingredient in many of the wound dressings described (Atta, 1999; Feldman and Goodrich, 1999; Ovington, 2002). In the Ebers Papyrus (1550 BC), the basic wound dressing used for numerous topical applications consisted of lint (vegetable fibres), grease (animal fat), and honey (Majno, 1975; Ovington, 2002). Honey was incorporated in many other prescriptions, including skin ointments, remedies for diseases of the eye, traumatic wound dressings, surgical dressings (including those used after circumcision), therapeutics inserted into the vulva for various diseases of the uterus and suppositories. Honey was also used to treat abscesses, suppurating sores, skin conditions due to scurvy, mouth ulcers, nail infections, ear infections, respiratory ailments, diabetes mellitus and diseases of the gut (Crane, 1999; Darby *et al*, 1977; Majno, 1975).

The Ancient Egyptians are just one example of a society that used honey extensively as a medicine. Beekeeping and the therapeutic use of honey spread from the Egyptians to many other cultures, and also evolved separately in other societies. The ailments treated with honey were as diverse as the cultures that used it, and include anything from insect bites to war wounds. *Table 1.1* provides some examples of the peoples that used honey medicinally.

Honey has always been popular as a wound dressing. It is now well established that keeping wounds moist will aid healing. However, this can have consequences for infection, which is a major factor in morbidity and mortality associated with wounds. The application of honey to a wound produces and maintains a moist environment and, as discussed in the following chapters, the antibacterial properties

Table 1.1: Some examples of the therapeutic use of honey by different cultures throughout history

People	Medicinal uses of honey	References
Anglo-Saxons	Eye diseases; 'dirty' and internal wounds; infected and chronic ulcers; removal of scabs; tumours; wounds resulting from amputation; reducing exudate	Crane, 1999; Naylor, 1999
Arabs	Burns; diseases of the eye, skin, and gut; fever; haemorrhoids; respiratory aliments	Ransome, 1937; Lev, 2003
Byzantines	Pharyngitis; throat abscesses; tinnitus; tonsillitis; ulcers of the ears	Ramoutsaki *et al*, 2000; Ramoutsaki *et al*, 2002
Chinese	Smallpox lesions to reduce scars ; wounds	Beck, 1938; Fu *et al*, 2001
Egyptians	Abscesses; diabetes mellitus; diseases of the ear, eye, and gut; gynaecological conditions; mouth ulcers; nail infections; respiratory ailments; skin conditions due to scurvy; suppurating sores; surgical dressings (including post circumcision); wound dressings	Majno, 1975; Atta, 1999; Crane, 1999; Feldman and Goodrich, 1999; Ovington, 2002
Finns	Wounds	Beck, 1938
Germans	Wounds	Crane, 1999
Greeks	Poisoning; respiratory aliments; wound dressings, particularly for infected wounds; ulcers; animal bites; head lice	Beck, 1938; Majno, 1975
Indians	Burns; constipation; eye and respiratory infections; internal disorders; wounds; ulcers	Ransome, 1937; Joshi and Godbole, 1970; Majno, 1975; Bibbings, 1984; Crane, 1999
Mexicans, Brazilians and other South American cultures	Gynaecological conditions; oral mycosis; infectious respiratory diseases; asthma; inflammation of the throat; antihelminthic actions; wounds and burns; ulcers; snake and rabid dog bites; cataract glaucoma and pterygium; as a tonic and to thin the blood	Ott, 1998; Costa-Neto, 2002; Alves and Rosa, 2006
Romans	Aches and ulcers of the ears; wound dressing; chronic ulcers	Beck, 1938; Majno, 1975; Crane, 1999
Sudanese	Cough suppressant; appetiser and stomach tonic; gastric ulcers; liver and gastrointestinal disorders; wounds	El-Kamali, 2000

of honey clear and prevent infection. This may explain much of the popularity of honey in wound dressings throughout the history of medicine. Often when honey was prescribed as a therapeutic agent, the type and/or location and/or time of collection was specified (Crane, 1999; Joshi and Godbole, 1970; Naylor, 1999; Ott, 1998). This indicates that many people were aware that the floral source of honey affected its medicinal properties.

Modern wound care

Although honey had a long history of medicinal use, it largely fell from favour during the era of modern antibiotic medicine. In the late 1960s and early 1970s the success of these drugs generated the misconception that infectious diseases had been conquered. In 1969 the US Surgeon General said, 'The time has come to close the book on infectious disease' (Nelson, 2003) — a statement that has proved to be rather premature. Infectious diseases are currently the third leading cause of death in the United States and the second leading cause of death worldwide (Spellberg *et al*, 2004). The rapid development and spread of antibiotic resistance among microorganisms contributes significantly to this.

Alarmingly, resistance has developed to every antibiotic introduced into clinical practice (Payne *et al*, 2007). Today, most bacteria that cause infections in hospitals are resistant to one or more antibiotics (Levy and Marshall, 2004), and some bacterial pathogens are resistant to all commonly employed antibacterial drugs (Paterson, 2006). Wound infections caused by drug-resistant organisms are common, and lead to increased costs, morbidity and mortality. There is an urgent need for new antibiotics with novel modes of action. However, few are currently under development (Spellberg *et al*, 2008). Many pharmaceutical companies have abandoned antimicrobial research as the cost of bringing new drugs to market is not being recovered, in part because microorganisms rapidly develop resistance to new products (Payne *et al*, 2007) .

It is possible that the problems associated with antibiotic-resistance and infection control have led to an increase in seeking effective non-antibiotic drug treatments. In the past few years there have been a rising number of *in vitro* and *in vivo* investigations into the antimicrobial and wound healing properties of honey, and many of these will be discussed in the following chapters.

References

Alves RRN, Rosa IL (2006) From cnidarians to mammals: The use of animals as remedies in fishing communities in NE Brazil. _J Ethnopharmacol_ **107**: 259–76

Atta HM (1999) Edwin Smith Surgical Papyrus: the oldest known surgical treatise. _Am Surgeon_ **65**: 1190–2

Beck BF (1938) _Honey and Health. A nutrimental, medicinal and historical commentary._ RM McBride & Co, New York

Bibbings J (1984) Honey, lizard dung and pigeons' blood. _Nurs Times_ **80**: 36–8

Costa-Neto EM (2002) The use of insects in folk medicine in the State of Bahia, northeastern Brazil, with notes on insects reported elsewhere in Brazilian folk medicine. _Human Ecol_ **30**: 245–63

Crane E (1986) Rock-paintings related to honey hunting. _Bee World_ **67**: 23–5

Crane E (1999) _The World History of Beekeeping and Honey Hunting._ Duckworth, London

Crane E (2001) _The Rock Art of Honey Hunters._ International Bee Research Association, Cardiff, UK

Darby WJ, Ghalioungui P, Grivetti L (1977) _Food: The Gift of Osiris._ Academic Press, London

El-Kamali HH (2000) Folk medicinal use of some animal products in Central Sudan. _J Ethnopharmacol_ **72**: 279–82

Feldman RP, Goodrich JT (1999) The Edwin Smith Surgical Papyrus. _Child's Nervous System_ **15**. 281–4

Fu XB, Wang ZG, Sheng ZY (2001) Advances in wound healing research in China: From antiquity to the present. _Wound Rep Regen_ **9**: 2–10

Joshi CG, Godbole NN (1970) The composition and medical properties of a natural honey as described in Ayurveda. _Indian Bee J_ **32**: 77–8.

Lev E (2003) Traditional healing with animals (zootherapy): medieval to present-day Levantine practice. _J Ethnopharmacol_ **85**: 107–18

Levy SB, Marshall B (2004) Antibacterial resistance worldwide: causes, challenges and responses. _Nature Med_ **10**: S122–S129

Majno G (1975) _The Healing Hand: man and wound in the ancient world._ Harvard University Press, Cambridge, Mass

Naylor IL (1999) Ulcer care in the Middle Ages. _J Wound Care_ **8**: 208–12

Nelson R (2003) Antibiotic development pipeline runs dry — new drugs to fight resistant organisms are not being developed, experts say. _Lancet_ **362**: 1726–7

Ott J (1998) The Delphic bee: bees and toxic honeys as pointers to psychoactive and other medicinal plants. _Economic Botany_ **52**: 260–6

Ovington LG (2002) The evolution of wound management: ancient origins and advances of the past 20 years. _Home Healthcare Nurse_ **20**: 652–6

Paterson DL (2006) The epidemiological profile of infections with multidrug-resistant *Pseudomonas aeruginosa* and *Acinetobacter* species. *Clin Infect Dis* **43**: S43–S48

Payne DJ, Gwynn MN, Holmes DJ, Pompliano DL (2007) Drugs for bad bugs: confronting the challenges of antibacterial discovery. *Nature Reviews Drug Discovery* **6**: 29–40

Ramoutsaki IA, Papadakis CE, Ramoutsakis JA, Helidonis ES (2000) Otolaryngologic diseases and medical treatment during the Byzantine period. *J Otolaryngol* **29**: 382–5

Ramoutsaki IA, Papadakis CE, Ramoutsakis IA, Helidonis ES (2002) Therapeutic methods used for otolaryngological problems during the Byzantine period. *Ann Otol Rhinol Laryngol* **111**: 553–7

Ransome HM (1937) *The Sacred Bee in Ancient Times and Folklore*. George Allen & Unwin Ltd, London

Spellberg B, Powers JH, Brass EP, Miller LG, Edwards JE (2004) Trends in antimicrobial drug development: Implications for the future. *Clin Infect Dis* **38**: 1279–86

Spellberg B, Guidos R, Gilbert D, Bradley J, Boucher HW, Scheld WM, *et al* (2008) The epidemic of antibiotic-resistant infections: A call to action for the medical community from the Infectious Diseases Society of America. *Clin Infect Dis* **46**: 155–64

Chapter 2

Why honey works

Peter Molan

There is increasing interest in using honey in wound care, but because there is relatively little promotion of honey products for wound care there is a common misconception that there is little evidence to support its use. However, there is in fact far more clinical evidence for the effectiveness of honey than there is for the myriad of modern wound dressings which are heavily advertised (Vermeulen *et al*, 2005). A review of the higher-level evidence for honey (Molan, 2006) revealed a great deal of evidence giving positive results for the use of honey in wound care. Since then, 16 more randomised controlled trials of honey have been published (Nagane *et al*, 2004; Okany *et al*, 2004; Bangroo *et al*, 2005; Johnson *et al*, 2005; Marshall *et al*, 2005; Okeniyi *et al*, 2005; Ingle *et al*, 2006; Mashhood *et al*, 2006; McIntosh and Thomson, 2006; Moolenaar *et al*, 2006; Tahmaz *et al*, 2006; Güneş and Eşer, 2007; Mphande *et al*, 2007; Nilforoushzadeh *et al*, 2007; Gethin and Cowman, 2008b; Jull *et al*, 2008) giving the sum of 33 randomised controlled trials involving a total of 3289 participants. The review (Molan, 2006) also summarised the details of five other forms of clinical trials with 97 patients treated with honey, and ten reports of studies of case series (totalling 276 cases), most of which were chronic wounds which healed after being treated with honey.

Although the catch-cry these days is evidence-based medicine, this vast amount of evidence is not sufficient to persuade many clinicians to try using honey. The reason for this has long been present in the medical profession. In 1830, a lament was published by John Renton in the *Edinburgh Medical and Surgical Journal* (34: 101):

> *When no satisfactory explanation can be afforded of the modus operandi of the agent, professional persons, unhappily for the*

interests of medical science, are too apt to reason upon the authenticity of the facts averred, instead of adopting the more simple and direct method of determining their value by subjecting them to the fact of further experience.

This chapter has been written to afford a satisfactory explanation of the '*modus operandi*' of honey; to explain biochemically why honey appears to be effective in bringing about rapid healing of wounds.

Formation and composition of honey

Nectar (or occasionally sap) is collected by foraging worker bees and delivered to the hive, where 'house bees' concentrate the harvested watery sugar solution by drying it in the warm draught created by multitudinous bees flapping their wings and generating heat by their 'aerobics'. During the intake of the nectar into the bees' crops, and subsequent regurgitation, enzymes are added by secretion from the hypopharyngeal gland which will help preserve the nectar. One of these enzymes, invertase, breaks sucrose (the principle sugar in nectar) into glucose and fructose, giving a mixture which is much more soluble than sucrose. The saturated or supersaturated solution of these two sugars has a sufficiently high osmolarity when honey is fully dried (i.e. to a point where it is about 17% water) to prevent the growth of any microorganisms.

Another enzyme added, glucose oxidase, generates hydrogen peroxide from the oxidation of glucose, and this serves to sterilise the nectar while it is being turned into honey. The other product of this enzymic reaction is gluconic acid, which gives honey a pH in the region of 3.5 to 4.5. This enzyme becomes inactive once the water content of the honey becomes low, but it will become active again if honey gets diluted. It is at maximal activity when honey is diluted to a concentration of about 50% (Bang, 2003).

Some of the other bee proteins added from the hypopharyngeal gland secretion also have bioactivity of relevance to wound healing (*Chapter 14*). Different types of honey will vary little in respect to their content of these various bee proteins. However, there is great variety in their content of different phytochemicals (plant chemicals), which, often occurring in trace quantities, give the different types of honey their characteristic colours, flavours, aromas, and bioactivities, such as antioxidant and anti-inflammatory properties (Molan, 1996). Being a concentrated plant fluid (nectar or sap), honey is basically a 'herbal medicine' with some bee proteins added. Herbal medicines are well known to be derived from different types of plants and produce medicines medicines with different therapeutic properties (Villegas _et al_, 1997).

Nutritional value of honey

As flowering plants have co-evolved with pollinating insects, the nectar they produce has to provide the nutrients necessary to ensure the survival of the pollinators. Honey contains a wide range of nutritional minerals, amino acids and vitamins (Haydak, 1975; White, 1975), although its precise composition varies depending on the floral source. It has been reported that wounds heal faster if a nutrient mixture is applied topically (Kaufman, 1984; Niinikoski, 1977; Silvetti, 1981; Viljanto, 1976), and honey, used as a wound dressing, will provide cells in the wound bed with such a nutrient mixture.

Honey can also promote healing by supplying glucose to keratinocytes, which require an energy source to migrate across the surface of a wound during reepithelialisation (Silver, 1980). The level of glucose in wound fluid of chronic wounds is low (Schultz, 2003). Honey is 30–40% glucose in its composition.

The sugars in honey provide an energy source for cells in the wound environment that remove bacteria and non-viable tissue and initiate the cascade of cytokines and growth factors that regulate healing (Tonks _et al_, 2003). Glycolysis is the major mechanism for energy production in macrophages, and depends on adequate levels which may be limited in areas surrounding the wound where capillaries have been damaged. Glycolysis is the only means by which cells obtain energy in the absence of oxygen; thus, the supply of sugar from honey allows macrophages to function well in damaged tissues where oxygen supply is often poor (Ryan and Majno, 1977).

In individuals with diabetes, the shortage of insulin leads to impaired glucose uptake into cells and this may be a factor that contributes to their characteristically poor wound healing (Edmonds, 2008) (_Chapter 8_). High glucose levels in a wound will establish the diffusion gradient across cell membranes, and thus enhance the entry of glucose by diffusion which is independent of the insulin-controlled active transport mechanism.

Bacteria always metabolise glucose in preference to amino acids. In the absence of glucose, malodorous sulphur compounds, amines and ammonia arise from the anaerobic bacterial metabolism of amino acids formed from the digestion of proteins in wound fluid, however, in the presence of glucose these are not formed (Nychas *et al*, 1988). This accounts for the rapid deodorising effect of honey in wounds, prior to the inhibitory effects of honey.

Osmotic action of honey

Osmosis is the movement of water across a membrane towards a concentrated solution. Solutions of high osmolarity cause removal of water molecules from cells. The outflow of lymph created by the osmotic action of honey is beneficial to the healing process.

The rate-limiting factor for growth of granulation tissue is the availability of oxygen (Silver, 1980). The surface area of a wound bed is too small to allow atmospheric oxygen to dissolve at a sufficient rate to supply cellular needs. In the lungs the vast surface area of the alveoli allows oxygen to be absorbed and bound to haemoglobin at a high rate. It is then distributed to cells in tissues by blood. Within a wound, irregularities in the capillaries supplying blood, limit the availability of oxygen. The presence of inflammation and concomitant oedema exacerbates this situation. The osmotically induced outflow of lymph from underlying tissue by the addition of honey promotes extra oxygenation. This outflow of lymph also provides an improved supply of nutrients to the growing cells on the wound surface. Furthermore, it flushes away proteases which may be inhibiting the repair process (see below). These benefits have also been demonstrated with topical negative pressure (TNP).

The osmotic action of honey also gives a moist healing environment without promoting bacterial growth if honeys of proven antibacterial activity are used. Provided there is sufficient honey present, its osmotic effects allow the presence of sufficient fluids to prevent the dressing adhering to the wound bed. It is also likely that honey activates proteolytic action which digests any fibrin clot (Molan, 2001). Thus, the presence of honey next to the wound bed helps to prevent pain at dressing changes and trauma to the newly-formed wound tissue.

Acidity of honey aids wound healing

The level of dissolved oxygen is a rate-limiting factor for fibroblast growth. Haemoglobin passing through the capillaries releases only about 25% of the oxygen it carries if the pH is at the normal blood level (7.4). However, if the pH drops to just 6.8, more than 50% of the oxygen carried is released. It has been observed that acidification of wounds speeds the rate of healing (Kaufman, 1985; Leveen, 1973). An alkaline pH is associated with wounds which are not healing, whereas an acidic pH is associated with healing (_Chapter 9_).

Acidification of wounds may also aid healing by decreasing protease activity which may be preventing wound healing by digesting the extracellular matrix and growth factors which are essential for tissue repair (see below). As discussed in _Chapter 9_, the proteases in wounds work best at neutral to alkaline pH values.

Thus, the acidity of honey is of benefit in wound treatment even though it sometimes causes pain where nocioceptor nerve endings, which detect heat and acidity, have become sensitised by factors produced in inflamed wound tissue.

Antioxidants

Honey contains a high level of antioxidants (Frankel, 1998; Gheldof, 2002; Gheldof, 2002; Gheldof, 2003; Henriques, 2006; Meda, 2005; Vela, 2007; Aljadi, 2004; Al-Mamary, 2002; D'Arcy, 2005; Blasa, 2006). After honey is ingested its antioxidants give protection in the bloodstream and within cells (Schramm, 2003).

Antioxidants neutralise free radicals, which are highly reactive molecules that are damaging to vitally important components of wound tissue such as proteins, cellular DNA and cell membranes. A large amount of free radical production occurs in wounds as a result of phagocytosis. When bacteria or necrotic cells are engulfed by phagocytes, an enzyme in the cell membrane becomes activated and produces the superoxide free radical. This in turn gives rise to hydrogen peroxide and other free radicals which are collectively known as 'reactive oxygen species' (ROS). Hydrogen peroxide is not included in this term, but it can diffuse out of the phagocytes and generate free radicals outside the cell. The superoxide radical is highly reactive and, although it can cross cell membranes, it usually reacts immediately before diffusion.

The chemical attractant is not hydrogen peroxide itself but a peptide produced from complement factor C5 in serum by oxidation by ROS free radicals (Shingu, 1984). This oxidation reaction would be inhibited by antioxidants. The attraction of neutrophils which results from the superoxide produced is similarly not a direct attraction to superoxide itself. The superoxide produced reacts with lipids in serum to create the attractant molecules (Flohé, 1985).

Manuka honey is unusual in containing a high level of methyl syringate, an antioxidant which neutralises the superoxide radical (Inoue, 2005). It also has another unusual type of antioxidant activity. This functions by binding iron and making it incapable of catalysing the formation of the extremely damaging hydroxide radical from hydrogen peroxide (Brangoulo and Molan, unpublished work). This iron-catalysed breakdown of hydrogen peroxide is considered to be a major source of free radical damage in the body (Puntarulo, 2005).

Far greater damage to tissues is caused by the activation of proteases in the wound tissues, than by the ROS themselves (Weiss *et al*, 1985; Ossanna *et al*, 1986; Peppin and Weiss, 1986). These protein-digesting enzymes are normally present in an inactive form (in the case of the matrix metalloproteases), or are kept inactive by the presence of an inhibitor (in the case of the neutrophil serine protease). The matrix metalloproteases are activated by oxidation (Van Wart, 1990) and the inhibitor of neutrophil protease in wound tissue is inactivated by oxidation (Flohé, 1985). Once activated, these proteases can destroy wound tissue. Thus, a wound can become ulcerated and a partial-thickness burn can become full-thickness if there is excessive production of ROS.

Activated proteases destroy both cytokines and tissue growth factors, that have essential regulatory functions. They also destroy the extracellular matrix, which are important for cellular attachment during migration and multiplication. The antioxidant activity of honey could thus be responsible for major protection of wound tissue where inflammation has caused an influx of phagocytes. In a clinical trial it was found that honey dressings prevented partial-thickness burns from converting to full-thickness burns which would have needed plastic surgery (Subrahmanyam, 1998). From the results of another clinical trial of honey dressings on burns, in which oxidative stress was measured, it was concluded that control of free radicals by the antioxidant action of honey was the way in which honey initiates healing in burns (Subrahmanyam, 2003).

Anti-inflammatory action

Excessive inflammation is the scourge of wound healing. A mild, short-lived state of inflammation is required to initiate the healing process, but when it becomes excessive the number of neutrophils and macrophages present increases and the ROS from their phagocytic activity cause damage which slows or prevents healing. If bacteria or any other trigger for inflammation persist, a chronic wound can result because of the activated proteases digesting cytokines, growth factors and extracellular matrix.

The large number of clinical reports where honey was shown to relieve the symptoms of inflammation has been reviewed (Molan, 2002). Some of these reports make it clear that this is not due simply to the clearance of the bacteria present, as decreased inflammation resulting from application of honey was seen in trials conducted with animals with experimentally inflicted wounds in which there were few or no bacteria present (Burlando, 1978; El-Banby, 1989; Gupta, 1992; Kandil, 1987; Kumar, 1993; Oryan, 1998; Postmes, 1997). The anti-inflammatory effect of honey was observed in studies on induced colitis in laboratory animals (Bilsel, 2002; Mahgoub, 2002) and in the wrist-joint stiffness test in guinea-pigs, which is a standard test for anti-inflammatory activity (Church, 1954).

The antibacterial activity of honey (*Chapter* 3) plays an important part in decreasing inflammation in wounds, as components of the cell wall of bacteria are potent stimulators of the inflammatory response (*Chapter* 14). The presence of slough in wounds also acts as an inflammatory stimulus and its removal following topical application of honey to wounds (Efem, 1988; Gethin and Cowman, 2008a) is another anti-inflammatory effect (*Chapter* 9).

The inflammatory response itself can set up a vicious cycle if the inflammatory stimulus is prolonged and superoxide and hydrogen peroxide are continuously produced because they act to recruit more neutrophils by chemical attraction (Flohé, 1985; Klyubin, 1996) (*Figures* 2.1 and 2.2). Hydrogen peroxide activates neutrophils, via the activation of the nuclear transcription factor NF-kB, to switch on genes to produce cytokines which amplify the inflammatory response by recruiting and activating leukocytes (Baeuerle, 1996). The recruited neutrophils in turn produce more hydrogen peroxide. Thus, there is a feed-back amplification of the inflammatory response, which exists while the stimulus continues.

With this being a cycle, hydrogen peroxide from other sources can trigger it. This explains why reperfusion injury gives rise to inflammation because the hydrogen peroxide is generated by cellular metabolism when the oxygen supply is restored after circulation-restricting pressure is relieved. It results in the formation of pressure and varicose ulcers. It has been shown that the oxidative species formed from hydrogen peroxide, rather than hydrogen peroxide itself, are responsible for activating NF-kB. Antioxidants prevent this activation (Grimble, 1994), therefore, honeys that contain antioxidants ame-liorate this effect (Schreck, 1991).

The ability of honey to neutralise free radicals has been demonstrated (van den Berg, 2008; Henriques, 2006). Clinically it has been shown that application of antioxidants to burns (Tanaka, 1995) and to corneal ulcers (Alio, 1995) decreases inflammation. However, recent research has revealed that honey also has another mechanism of anti-inflammatory activity, as it directly inhibits the process of phagocytosis itself, thus preventing oxygen free radicals being formed in the first place (Bean, A; University of Waikato, personal communication). In the author's opinion, it is most likely that both mechanisms are involved. Although it may

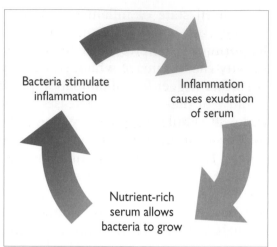

Figure 2.1: The vicious cycle that can result when bacteria are in a wound. It can be started by infection or by inflammation resulting from other causes

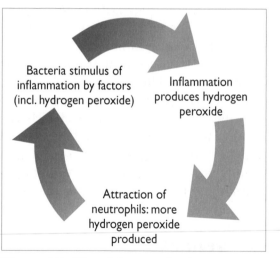

Figure 2.2: The vicious cycle that can result from feed-back amplification of the inflammatory response by the hydrogen peroxide that is produced

be thought that the antioxidant action neutralising free radicals would be more important once inflammation has become established, it must be remembered that in the vicious cycle there is ongoing phagocytosis. Inhibition of this would help break the cycle.

Both the prevention of free radical formation and the quenching of free radicals are important factors in the ability of honey to minimise hypertrophic scarring. The ROS formed in inflammation stimulate the activity of the fibroblasts which produce the collagen fibres of scar tissue, and in situations where there is prolonged inflammation, their over-stimulation can lead to hypergranulation and fibrosis (Murrell, 1990). Like with the stimulation of leukocytes, this is via oxidation of NF-kB and can be inhibited by antioxidants (Murrell, 1990). There have been numerous clinical reports of this therapeutic feature of honey (Dunford _et al_, 2000; Efem, 1993; Subrahmanyam, 1991; Subrahmanyam, 1994). Free radicals have been implicated in hypertrophic scar formation following burn injuries (Wan, 1999).

Immunostimulatory activity

It may be thought that the removal of the impediments to healing by way of the antibacterial, antioxidant and anti-inflammatory actions of honey would account for the rapid rate of healing brought about by honey, and the 'jump-start' of healing in wounds where healing has stalled (Molan, 2002). But there is evidence from studies on experimental wounds in animals that honey stimulates the growth of repair tissues. A study on mice found that honey gave a 114% increase in the extent of epithelialisation and a 69% increase in the thickness of granulation tissue compared with a saline control (Bergman, 1983). Stimulation of angiogenesis by honey has been observed histologically (Gupta, 1992; Kumar, 1993). The most likely mechanism for such promotion of growth is the stimulation of cytokine production by honey, which is covered in _Chapter 14_.

References _____

Al-Mamary M, Al-Meeri A, Al-Habori M (2002) Antioxidant activities and total phenolics of different types of honey. _Nutrition Res_ 22(9): 1041–7

Alio JL, Ayala MJ, Mulet ME, Artola A, Ruiz JM, Bellot J (1995) Antioxidant therapy in the treatment of experimental acute corneal inflammation. _Ophthalmic Res_ 27(3): 136–43

Aljadi AM, Kamaruddin MY (2004) Evaluation of the phenolic contents and antioxidant capacities of two Malaysian floral honeys. _Food Chem_ 85(4): 513–8

Baeuerle PA, Rupec RA, Pahl HL (1996) Reactive oxygen intermediates as second messengers of a general pathogen response. *Pathol Biol (Paris)* 44(1): 29–35

Bang LM, Buntting C, Molan PC (2003) The effect of dilution on the rate of hydrogen peroxide production in honey and its implications for wound healing. *J Altern Complement Med* 9(2): 267–73

Bangroo AK, Katri R, Chauhan S (2005) Honey dressing in pediatric burns. *J Indian Assoc Pediatr Surg* 10(3): 172–5

Bergman A, Yanai J, Weiss J, Bell D, David MP (1983) Acceleration of wound healing by topical application of honey. An animal model. *Am J Surg* 145: 374–6

Bilsel Y, Bugra D, Yamaner S, Bulut T, Cevikbas U, Turkoglu U (2002) Could honey have a place in colitis therapy? Effects of honey, prednisolone, and disulfiram on inflammation, nitric oxide, and free radical formation. *Dig Surg* 19: 306–12

Blasa M, Candiracci M, Accorsi A, Piacentini MP, Albertini MC, Piatti E (2006) Raw Millefiori honey is packed full of antioxidants. *Food Chem* 97(2): 217–22

Burlando F (1978) Sull'azione terapeutica del miele nelle ustioni. *Minerva Dermatol* 113: 699–706

Chirife J, Scarmato G, Herszage L (1982) Scientific basis for use of granulated sugar in treatment of infected wounds. *Lancet* i(March 6): 560–1

Church J (1954) Honey as a source of the anti-stiffness factor. *Fed Proc Am Physiol Soc* 13(1): 26

D'Arcy BR (2005) *Antioxidants in Australian floral honeys — identification of health-enhancing nutrient components*. Report for the Rural Industries Research and Development Corporation, Australia: 1–84

Dunford C, Cooper R, Molan PC (2000) Using honey as a dressing for infected skin lesions. *Nurs Times* 96(14 NT-plus): 7–9

Edmonds MA (2008) Natural history and framework for managing diabetic foot ulcers. *Br J Nurs* 17(11): S20, S22, S24–9

Efem SE (1988) Clinical observations on the wound healing properties of honey. *Br J Surg* 75(7): 679–81

Efem SE (1993) Recent advances in the management of Fournier's gangrene: Preliminary observations. *Surgery* 113(2): 200–4

Efem SE (1988) Clinical observations on the wound healing properties of honey. *Br J Surg* 75(7): 679–81

El-Banby M, Kandil A, Abou-Sehly G, El-Sherif ME, Abdel-Wahed K (1989) *Healing effect of floral honey and honey from sugar-fed bees on surgical wounds (animal model)*. Fourth International Conference on Apiculture in Tropical Climates, Cairo, International Bee Research Association, London

Flohé L, Beckmann R, Giertz H, Loschen G (1985) Oxygen-centred free radicals as mediators of inflammation. In: Sies H, ed. *Oxidative Stress*. Academic Press, London, Orlando: 403–35

Frankel S, Robinson GE, Berenbaum MR (1998) Antioxidant capacity and correlated characteristics of 14 unifloral honeys. *J Apic Res* 37(1): 27–31

Gethin G, Cowman S (2008a) Bacteriological changes in sloughy leg ulcers treated with manuka honey or hydrogel: an RCT. _J Wound Care_ 17(6): 241–4, 246–7

Gethin G, Cowman S (2008b) Manuka honey vs. hydrogel — a prospective, open label, multicentre, randomised controlled trial to compare desloughing efficacy and healing outcomes in venous ulcers. _J Clin Nurs._ Aug 23. [Epub ahead of print]

Gheldof N, Engeseth NJ (2002) Antioxidant capacity of honeys from various floral sources based on the determination of oxygen radical absorbance capacity and inhibition of _in vitro_ lipoprotein oxidation in human serum samples. _J Agric Food Chem_ 50(10): 3050–5

Gheldof N, Wang X-H, Engeseth NJ (2002) Identification and quantification of antioxidant components of honeys from various floral sources. _J Agric Food Chem_ 50: 5870–7

Gheldof N, Wang X-H, Engeseth NJ (2003) Buckwheat honey increases serum antioxidant capacity in humans. _J Agric Food Chem_ 51(5): 1500–5

Grimble GF (1994) Nutritional antioxidants and the modulation of inflammation: theory and practice. _New Horizons_ 2(2): 175–85

Güneş ÜY, Eşer I (2007) Effectiveness of a honey dressing for healing pressure ulcers. _J Wound Ostomy Continence Nurs_ 34(2): 184–90

Gupta SK, Singh H, Varshney AC, Prakash P (1992) Therapeutic efficacy of honey in infected wounds in buffaloes. _Indian J Anim Sci_ 62(6): 521–3

Haydak MH, Crane E, Duisberg H, Gochnauer TA, Morse RA, White JW, Wix P (1975) _Biological Properties of Honey_ London, Heinemann.

Henriques A, Jackson S, Cooper R, Burton N (2006) Free radical production and quenching in honeys with wound healing potential. _J Antimicrob Chemother_ 58(4): 773–7

Ingle R, Levin J, Polinder K (2006) Wound healing with honey — a randomised controlled trial. _S Afr Med J_ 96(9): 831–5

Inoue K, Murayama S, Seshimo F, Takeba K, Yoshimura YHN (2005) Identification of phenolic compound in manuka honey as specific superoxide anion radical scavenger using electron spin resonance (ESR) and liquid chromatography with coulometric array detection. _J Sci Food Agric_ 85(5): 872–8

Johnson DW, van Eps C, Mudge DW, Wiggins KJ, Armstrong K, Hawley CM, _et al_ (2005) Randomized, controlled trial of topical exit-site application of honey (Medihoney) versus mupirocin for the prevention of catheter-associated infections in hemodialysis patients. _J Am Soc Nephrol_ 16(5): 1456–62

Jull A, Walker N, Parag V, Molan P, Rodgers A (2008) Randomized clinical trial of honey-impregnated dressings for venous leg ulcers. _Br J Surg_ 95(2): 175–82

Kandil A, El-Banby M, Abdel-Wahed K, Abou-Sehly G, Ezzat N (1987) Healing effect of true floral and false nonfloral honey on medical wounds. _J Drug Res (Cairo)_ 17(1–2): 71–5

Kaufman T, Eichenlaub EH, Angel MF, Levin M, Futrell JW (1985) Topical acidification promotes healing of experimental deep partial-thickness skin burns: a randomised double-blind preliminary study. *Burns* 12: 84–90

Kaufman T, Levin M, Hurwitz DJ (1984) The effect of topical hyperalimentation on wound healing rate and granulation tissue formation of experimental deep second degree burns in guinea-pigs. *Burns* 10(4): 252–6

Klyubin IV, Kirpichnikova KM, Gamaley IA (1996) Hydrogen peroxide-induced chemotaxis of mouse peritoneal neutrophils. *Eur J Cell Biol* 70(4): 347–51

Kumar A, Sharma VK, Singh HP, Prakash P, Singh SP (1993) Efficacy of some indigenous drugs in tissue repair in buffaloes. *Indian Vet J* 70(1): 42–4

Leveen HH, Falk G, Borek B, Diaz C, Lynfield Y, Wynkoop BJ, *et al* (1973) Chemical acidification of wounds. An adjuvant to healing and the unfavourable action of alkalinity and ammonia. *Ann Surg* 178(6): 745–53

Mahgoub AA, el-Medany AH, Hagar HH, Sabah DM (2002) Protective effect of natural honey against acetic acid-induced colitis in rats. *Trop Gastroenterol* 23(2): 82–7

Marshall C, Queen J, Manjooran J (2005) Honey vs povidone iodine following toenail surgery. *Wounds UK* 1(1): 10, 14, 16–18

Mashhood AA, Khan TA, Sami AN (2006) Honey compared with 1% silver sulfadiazine cream in the treatment of superficial and partial thickness burns. *J Pak Assoc Dermatologists* 16(1): 14–19

McIntosh CD, Thomson CE (2006) Honey dressing versus paraffin tulle gras following toenail surgery. *J Wound Care* 15(3): 133–6

Meda A, Lamien CE, Romito M, Millogo J, Nacoulma OG (2005) Determination of the total phenolic, flavonoid and proline contents in Burkina Fasan honey, as well as their radical scavenging activity. *Food Chem* 91(3): 571–7

Molan PC (1996) Authenticity of honey. In: Ashurst PR, Dennis MJ, eds. *Food Authentication*. Blackie Academic and Professional, London: 259–303

Molan PC (2001) Why honey is effective as a medicine: The scientific explanation of its effects. *Bee World* 82(1): 22–40

Molan PC (2002) Re-introducing honey in the management of wounds and ulcers - theory and practice. *Ostomy/Wound Management* 48(11): 28–40

Molan PC (2006) The evidence supporting the use of honey as a wound dressing. *Int J Lower Extrem Wounds* 5(1): 40–54

Moolenaar M, Poorter RL, van der Toorn PP, Lenderink AW, Poortmans P, Egberts AC (2006) The effect of honey compared to conventional treatment on healing of radiotherapy-induced skin toxicity in breast cancer patients. *Acta Oncol* 45(5): 623–4

Mphande AN, Killowe C, Phalira S, Jones HW, Harrison WJ (2007) Effects of honey and sugar dressings on wound healing. *J Wound Care* 16(7): 317–9

Murrell GAC, Francis MJO, Bromley L (1990) Modulation of fibroblast proliferation by oxygen free radicals. *Biochem J* 265: 659–65

Nagane NS, Ganu JV, Bhagwat VR, Subramanium M (2004) Efficacy of topical honey therapy against silver sulphadiazine treatment in burns: A biochemical study. _Indian J Clin Biochem_ **19**(2): 173–6

Niinikoski J, Kivisaari J, Viljanto J (1977) Local hyperalimentation of experimental granulation tissue. _Acta Chem Scand_ **143**: 201–6

Nilforoushzadeh MA, Jaffary F, Moradi S, Derakhshan R, Haftbaradaran E (2007) Effect of topical honey application along with intralesional injection of glucantime in the treatment of the cutaneous leishmaniasis. _BMC Complement Altern Med_ **7**(1): 13–17

Nychas GJ, Dillon VM, Board RG (1988) Glucose, the key substrate in the microbiological changes in meat and certain meat products. _Biotechnol Appl Biochem_ **10**: 203–31

Okany CC, Atimomo CE, Akinyanju OO (2004) Efficacy of natural honey in the healing of leg ulcers in sickle cell anaemia. _Niger Postgrad Med J_ **11**(3): 179–81

Okeniyi JAO, Olubanjo OO, Ogunlesi TA, Oyelami OA (2005) Comparison of healing of incised abscess wounds with honey and EUSOL dressing. _J Altern Complement Med_ **11**(3): 511–13

Oryan A, Zaker SR (1998) Effects of topical application of honey on cutaneous wound healing in rabbits. _J Vet Med Ser_ **45**(3): 181–8

Postmes TJ, Bosch MMC, Dutrieux R, van Baare J, Hoekstra MJ (1997) Speeding up the healing of burns with honey. An experimental study with histological assessment of wound biopsies. In: Mizrahi A, Lensky Y, eds. _Bee Products: Properties, Applications and Apitherapy_. Plenum Press, New York: 27–37

Puntarulo S (2005) Iron, oxidative stress and human health. _Mol Aspects Med_ **26**(4–5): 299–312

Ryan GB, Majno G (1977) Acute inflammation: A review. _Am J Pathol_ **86**: 183–276

Schramm DD, Karim M, Schrader HR, Holt RR, Cardetti M, Keen CL (2003) Honey with high levels of antioxidants can provide protection to healthy human subjects. _J Agric Food Chem_ **51**(6): 1732–5

Schreck R, Rieber P, Baeuerle PA (1991) Reactive oxygen intermediates as apparently widely used messengers in the activation of the NF-kB transcription factor and HIV-1. _EMBO J_ **10**(8): 2247–58

Schultz GS, Sibbald RG, Falanga V, Ayello EA, Dowsett C, Harding K, _et al_ (2003) Wound bed preparation: a systematic approach to wound management. _Wound Rep Regen_ **11**(Suppl 1): S1–S28

Shingu M, Nobunaga M (1984) Chemotactic activity generated in human serum from the fifth component of complement by hydrogen peroxide. _Am J Pathol_ **117**(2): 201–6

Silver IA (1980) The physiology of wound healing. In: Hunt TK, ed. _Wound Healing and Wound Infection: theory and surgical practice_. Appleton-Century-Crofts, New York: 11–28

Silvetti AN, Krejci-Simmons C, Schwartz D (1981) Accelerated wound healing and infection control through the topical application of nutrients. *Fed Proc* **40**(3, Part II): 922 (Abstract no. 3929)

Subrahmanyam M (1991) Topical application of honey in treatment of burns. *Br J Surg* **78**(4): 497–8

Subrahmanyam M (1994) Honey-impregnated gauze versus amniotic membrane in the treatment of burns. *Burns* **20**(4): 331–3

Subrahmanyam M (1998) A prospective randomised clinical and histological study of superficial burn wound healing with honey and silver sulfadiazine. *Burns* **24**(2): 157–61

Subrahmanyam M, Sahapure AG, Nagane NS, Bhagwat VR, Ganu JV (2003) Free radical control — the main mechanism of the action of honey in burns. *Ann Burns Fire Disasters* **16**(3): 135–8

Tahmaz L, Erdemir F, Kibar Y, Cosar A, Yalcyn O (2006) Fournier's gangrene: Report of thirty-three cases and a review of the literature. *Int J Urol* **13**(7): 960–7

Tanaka H, Hanumadass M, Matsuda H, Shimazaki S, Walter RJ, Matsuda T (1995) Hemodynamic effects of delayed initiation of antioxidant therapy (beginning two hours after burn) in extensive third-degree burns. *J Burn Care Rehabil* **16**(6): 610–5

Tonks AJ, Cooper RA, Jones KP, Blair S, Parton J, Tonks A (2003) Honey stimulates inflammatory cytokine production from monocytes. *Cytokine* 7 **21**(5): 242–7

van den Berg AJ, van den Worm E, van Ufford HC, Halkes SB, Hoekstra MJ, Beukelman CJ (2008) An *in vitro* examination of the antioxidant and anti-inflammatory properties of buckwheat honey. *J Wound Care* **17**(4): 172–8

Van Wart HE, Birkedal-Hansen H (1990) The cysteine switch: A principle of regulation of metalloproteinase activity with potential applicability to the entire matrix metalloproteinase gene family. *Proc Nat Acad Sci USA* **87**(14): 5578–82

Vela L, de Lorenzo C, Pérez RA (2007) Antioxidant capacity of Spanish honeys and its correlation with polyphenol content and other physicochemical properties. *J Sci Food Agric* **87**(6): 1069–75

Vermeulen H, Ubbink DT, Goossens A, de Vos R, Legemate DA (2005) Systematic review of dressings and topical agents for surgical wounds healing by secondary intention. *Br J Surg* **92**(6): 665–72

Viljanto J, Raekallio j (1976) Local hyperalimentation of open wounds. *Br J Surg* **63**: 427–30

Villegas LF, Fernández ID, Maldonado H, Torres R, Zavaleta A, Vaisberg AJ, Hammond GB (1997) Evaluation of the wound-healing activity of selected traditional medicinal plants from Peru. *J Ethnopharmacol* **55**(3): 193–200

Wan KC, Evans JH (1999) Free radical involvement in hypertrophic scar formation. *Free Radic Biol Med* **26**(5–6): 603–8

White JW (1975) Composition of honey. In: Crane E, ed. *Honey: A Comprehensive Survey*. Heinemann, London: 157–206

CHAPTER 3

ANTIBACTERIAL ACTIVITY OF HONEY

Shona Blair

There have been numerous investigations into the antibacterial activity of honey. Over 50 different species of bacteria have been tested for their sensitivity to a wide variety of honeys, these investigations are summarised in *Table 3.1*. Multiple strains were often tested, as were many clinical isolates. In some cases, the minimum inhibitory concentration (MIC) was reported. The MIC is the lowest concentration of an antimicrobial that will inhibit visible growth of a microorganism, and it is the most commonly described parameter of antibacterial agents. The reported MICs ranged from 2–100% honey depending on the organism and the type of honey, as well as the method used. In many cases a control sugar solution was also tested, and it was usually found to possess a significantly lower inhibitory activity.

The results from many of the different authors investigating the antibacterial activity of honey cannot be directly compared as different methods were used, and the type of honey was often undefined and infrequently chosen for a standard level of activity. However, it is clear that many honeys exhibited significant, broad-spectrum antibacterial activity, even though the floral source affects the degree of this activity. The reports summarised in *Table 3.1* have been published over the past 30+ years. More recently there have been an increasing number of reports in this field, possibly partly due to our decreasing antibiotic arsenal as well as an increasing awareness of the medicinal efficacy of certain honeys.

The antibacterial activity of honey results from its high sugar content, low pH, enzymic production of hydrogen peroxide and extra, potent florally-derived factors in some honeys such as certain *Leptospermum* spp. from New Zealand and Australia, colloquially referred to as manuka and jelly bush respectively (Molan, 1992). Phenolic components have been shown to contribute in a minor way to the non-peroxide activity of *Leptospermum* honeys (Weston *et al*, 2000). Recently, it has been proposed that unusually high levels of methylglyoxal in these honeys accounts for the non-peroxide activity they possess (Adams *et al*, 2008; Mavric *et al*, 2008). However, this does not completely explain the non-peroxide activity of these *Leptospermum* honeys. Considering the MIC Mavric *et al* (2008) reported for methylgyoxal, and the levels of methylgyoxal they found in their manuka honey samples, this honey would be ineffective at low concentrations, which is not the case (Cooper *et al*, 1999; George and Cutting, 2007). Also, examination of the graph published by Adams *et al* (2008), showing the correlation between antibacterial activity and concentration of methylglyoxal reveals that it is linear at higher levels of activity, which would be pure manuka honey, and that extrapolation of this line to zero methylglyoxal leaves a substantial amount of activity unaccounted for by methylglyoxal.

The variation in the antibacterial activity of honey

Here we concentrate mainly on the honey produced by the European honey bee, *Apis mellifera*. This bee is most commonly used for commercial honey production as it yields high amounts of honey, will nest and produce honey in boxes designed for easy honey extraction and is reasonably easy to handle. However, there have been several reports of the antibacterial activity of honey from other bee species, and in many instances these honeys are still used by local indigenous people as part of their traditional medical practices (Wakhle and Desai, 1991; Martins *et al*, 1997; Garedew *et al*, 2003; Miorin *et al*, 2003; DeMera and Angert, 2004; Torres *et al*, 2004; Goncalves *et al*, 2005; Temaru *et al*, 2007; Irish *et al*, 2008). However, most commercial quantities of honey, including readily available medical grade ones, are produced by *Apis mellifera*.

Many of the ancients appreciated the fact that when bees visited different flowers, honeys with different medicinal properties arose. Today there is still a poor appreciation of the vast range in the antibacterial activity of honey. From a medical point of view, honey should not be viewed as a generic product. For example, in a survey

Table 3.1: Laboratory testing of honey samples using bacterial cultures		
Organism	Honey type	References
Acinetobacter spp.	Unspecified, Saudia Arabia Manuka	Ali et al, 1991 Kouda et al, 2004
Achromobacter	Six honeys from the West Indies of unspecified floral origin	James et al, 1972
Actinomyces pyogenes	_Leptospermum scoparium, Knightia excelsa_, New Zealand	Allen and Molan, 1997
Aeromonas hydrophilia	Trefoil, Egypt Unspecified, Nigeria	Wahdan, 1998 Obi et al, 1994
Bacillus cereus	Langnese, Germany 31 honeys, including some of Spanish origin Multi-floral Turkish honeys from different regions Buckwheat, tarweed, manuka, _Melaleuca_ and saw palmetto honeys	El-Sukhon et al, 1994 Gallardo-Chacon et al, 2008 Mercan et al, 2007 Mundo et al, 2004
Bacillus stearothermophilus	Buckwheat, Tarweed, Manuka, _Melaleuca_ and saw palmetto honeys	Mundo et al, 2004
Bacillus subtilis	Unspecified type and number of Egyptian honeys 15 unprocessed honey samples of unspecified floral origin from Sudan An unspecified number of honeys from Nigeria, one English, and one German honey were used to prepare honey distillates Six honeys from the West Indies of unspecified floral origin	Zaghloul et al, 2001 Farouk et al, 1988 Obaseiki-Ebor et al, 1983 James et al, 1972
Bacteroides fragilis	Unspecified, Nigeria	Efem et al, 1992
Bacteroides spp.	Unspecified, Egypt	Elbagoury and Rasmy, 1993
Brucella spp.	Unspecified, Saudi Arabia	Ali et al, 1991
Burkholderia cepacia	_Leptospermum scoparium_, pasture honey, New Zealand	Cooper et al, 2000
Campylobacter jejuni	Unspecified, Nigeria Nigerian honey	Obi et al, 1994 Adebolu, 2005
Citrobacter diversus	_Syzygium cumini_, India	Subrahmanyam et al, 2001

Table 3.1: Cont		
Citrobacter freundii	*Syzygium cumini*, India	Subrahmanyam *et al*, 2001
Clostridium botulinum	Lime honey, country unspecified, possibly the Netherlands	Postmes *et al*, 1993
Clostridium perfringens	Lime honey, country unspecified, possibly the Netherlands	Postmes *et al*, 1993
Clostridium tetani	Unspecified, Nigeria	Efem *et al*, 1992
Clostridium welchii	Unspecified, Nigeria	Efem *et al*, 1992
Corynebacterium diphtheriae	Six honeys from the West Indies of unspecified floral origin	James *et al*, 1972
Enterobacter spp.	Unspecified, Saudi Arabia Revamil, (Bfactory), a medical-grade honey of unspecified floral origin Melghat honey, India	Ali *et al*, 1991 Kwakman *et al*, 2008 Tambekar and Rathod, 2007
Enterococcus spp.	*Leptospermum scoparium*, Pasture honey, New Zealand Revamil, Bfactory, a medical-grade honey of unspecified floral origin Manuka	Cooper *et al*, 2002b Kwakman *et al*, 2008 Kouda *et al*, 2004
VRE	*Leptospermum scoparium*, Pasture honey, New Zealand Medihoney, a medical grade *Leptospermum* honey blend	Cooper *et al*, 2002b George and Cutting, 2007
Enterococcus faecalis	Unspecified, Nigeria Unspecified, South Africa 31 honeys, including some of Spanish origin Eucalyptus, lavender and chestnut honeys	Efem *et al*, 1992 Jeddar *et al*, 1985 Gallardo-Chacon *et al*, 2008 Wojtyczka *et al*, 2007
Escherichia coli	Unspecified, various honeys from Oman, Uganda, Tanzania, Nigeria and South Africa Coorg, Indian *Syzygium cumini*, India	Al-Jabri *et al*, 2003 Shamala *et al*, 2002 Subrahmanyam *et al*, 2001
	Coorg, Indian	Shamala *et al*, 2002
	Syzygium cumini, India	Subrahmanyam *et al*, 2001

Table 3.1: Cont		
Escherichia coli cont	Unprocessed buckwheat and blueberry, processed safflower, avocado and clover honeys	Taormina _et al_, 2001
	Unspecified type and number of Egyptian honeys	Zaghloul et _al_, 2001
	Artisan orange, industrial orange and artisan citrus honey, Italy	Sinigaglia _et al_, 2000
	Unspecified, Nigeria	Obi _et al_, 1994
	Lime, Acacia and fruit tree honey, country unspecified, possibly the Netherlands	Postmes _et al_, 1993
	Unspecified, Nigeria	Efem _et al_, 1992
	Leptospermum scoparium, Knightia excelsa, New Zealand	Willix _et al_, 1992
	Unspecified, Saudi Arabia	Ali _et al_, 1991
	15 unprocessed honey samples of unspecified floral origin from Sudan	Farouk _et al_, 1988
	Unspecified, South Africa	Jeddar _et al_, 1985
	Cotton, clover and orange, Egypt	Radwan _et al_, 1984
	An unspecified number of honeys from Nigeria, one English, and one German honey were used to prepare honey distillates	Obaseiki-Ebor _et al_, 1983
	Six honeys from the West Indies of unspecified floral origin	James _et al_, 1972
	Unspecified	Ott and Morris, 2008
	Revamil, (Bfactory), a medical-grade honey of unspecified floral origin	Kwakman _et al_, 2008
	31 honeys, including some of Spanish origin	Gallardo-Chacon _et al_, 2008
	Eucalyptus, lavender and chestnut honeys	Wojtyczka _et al_, 2007
	Melghat honey, India	Tambekar and Rathod, 2007
	Multi-floral Turkish honeys from different regions	Mercan _et al_, 2007

Table 3.1: *Cont*		
Escherichia coli cont	Iranian honey	Jalali *et al*, 2007
	Buenos Arian honeys	Fangio *et al*, 2007
	15 unspecified honeys, probably Argentinean	Basualdo *et al*, 2007
	Various honeys sourced from within Venezuela	Cabrera *et al*, 2006
	42 Canadian honeys	Brudzynski, 2006
	Lavender, manuka, paterson's curse, red stringy bark, rewa rewa, rosemary and Medihoney, a medical grade *Leptospermum* honey blend	Wilkinson and Cavanagh, 2005
	20 honeys from the Czech Republic	Vorlova *et al*, 2005
	25 Costa Rican honeys	Estrada *et al*, 2005
	10 Indian honeys	Amit *et al*, 2005
	Honey from United Arab Emirates	Al-Waili *et al*, 2005
	Saudi Arabian honeys	Al-Hindi, 2005
	Nigerian honey	Adebolu, 2005
	Buckwheat, Tarweed, manuka, *Melaleuca* and saw palmetto honeys	Mundo *et al*, 2004
	Multiple non-manuka honeys from New Zealand	Brady *et al*, 2004
	Ethiopian honeys	Andargachew *et al*, 2004
Helicobacter pylori	Roy freese, wildflower and clover from North America, creamed manuka from New Zealand	Osato *et al*, 1999
	Leptospermum scoparium, New Zealand	Al-Somal *et al*, 1994
	Unspecified, Saudi Arabia	Ali *et al*, 1991
	Chestnut, rhododendron and a multi-floral honey from Eastern Anatolia	Kucuk *et al*, 2007
Haemophilus influenzae	Trefoil, Egypt	Wahdan, 1998
	Unspecified, South Africa	Jeddar *et al*, 1985
Klebsiella pneumoniae	*Syzygium cumini*, India	Subrahmanyam *et al*, 2001
	Trefoil, Egypt	Wahdan, 1998

Table 3.1: *Cont*		
Klebsiella pneumoniae cont	*Leptospermum scoparium, Knightia excelsa,* New Zealand	Allen and Molan, 1997
	Unspecified, Nigeria	Efem *et al*, 1992
	Unspecified, South Africa	Jeddar *et al*, 1985
	Unspecified	Ott and Morris, 2008
	Melghat honey, India	Tambekar and Rathod, 2007
	15 Unspecified honeys, probably Argentinean	Basualdo *et al*, 2007
	Multi-floral Turkish honeys from different regions	Mercan *et al*, 2007
Klebsiella spp.	Unspecified type and number of Egyptian honeys	Zaghloul *et al*, 2001
	Local Agmark brand honey, Mumbai	Karayil *et al*, 1998
	Unspecified, Saudi Arabia	Ali *et al*, 1991
	15 unprocessed honey samples of unspecified floral origin from Sudan	Farouk *et al*, 1988
	An unspecified number of honeys from Nigeria, one English, and one German honey were used to prepare honey distillates	Obaseiki-Ebor *et al*, 1983
	Six honeys from the West Indies of unspecified floral origin	James *et al*, 1972
	Revamil, (Bfactory), a medical-grade honey of unspecified floral origin	Kwakman *et al*, 2008
	Ethiopian honeys	Andargachew *et al*, 2004
Lactobacillus acidophilus	Unspecified, Czech Republic	Curda and Plockova, 1995
	Buckwheat, tarweed, manuka,	Mundo *et al*, 2004
	Melaleuca, and saw palmetto honeys	Mundo *et al*, 2004
Lactococcus spp.	Unspecified, Czech Republic	Curda and Plockova, 1995
Listeria monocytogenes	Unprocessed buckwheat and blueberry, processed safflower, avocado and clover honeys	Taormina *et al*, 2001

Table 3.1: *Cont*		
Listeria monocytogenes cont	Unspecified, South Africa	Jeddar *et al*, 1985
	31 honeys, including some of Spanish origin	Gallardo-Chacon *et al*, 2008
	Various honeys sourced from within Venezuela	Cabrera *et al*, 2006
	20 honeys from the Czech Republic	Vorlova *et al*, 2005
	25 Costa Rican honeys	Estrada *et al*, 2005
	Acacia honey	Dugalic-Vrndic *et al*, 2005
	Saudi Arabian honeys	Al-Hindi, 2005
	Buckwheat, tarweed, manuka, *Melaleuca* and saw palmetto honeys	Mundo *et al*, 2004
Micrococcus spp.	Six honeys from the West Indies of unspecified floral origin	James *et al*, 1972
	Multi-floral Turkish honeys from different regions	Mercan *et al*, 2007
Neisseria spp.	Six honeys from the West Indies of unspecified floral origin	James *et al*, 1972
Nocardia asteroides	*Leptospermum scoparium, Knightia excelsa*, New Zealand	Allen and Molan, 1997
Plesiomonas shigelloides	Unspecified, Nigeria	Obi *et al*, 1994
Proteus spp.	Unspecified, Saudi Arabia	Ali *et al*, 1991
	6 honeys from the West Indies of unspecified floral origin	James *et al*, 1972
Proteus mirabilis	Syzygium cumini, India	Subrahmanyam *et al*, 2001
	Trefoil, Egypt	Wahdan, 1998
	Unspecified, Nigeria	Efem *et al*, 1992
	Knightia excelsa, Leptospermum scoparium, New Zealand	Willix *et al*, 1992
	Unspecified, South Africa	Jeddar *et al*, 1985
	An unspecified number of honeys from Nigeria, one English, and one German honey were used to prepare honey distillates	Obaseiki-Ebor *et al*, 1983

Table 3.1: *Cont*		
Proteus mirabilis cont	Unspecified	Ott and Morris, 2008
	Various honeys sourced from within Venezuela	Cabrera *et al*, 2006
	Ethiopian honeys	Andargachew *et al*, 2004
Proteus vulgaris	*Syzygium cumini*, India	Subrahmanyam *et al*, 2001
	Unspecified type and number of Egyptian honeys	Zaghloul *et al*, 2001
	Melghat honey, India	Tambekar and Rathod, 2007
	Ethiopian honey	Andargachew *et al*, 2004
Pseudomonas spp.	*Leptospermum scoparium*, pasture honey, New Zealand	Cooper and Molan, 1999
	Local Agmark brand honey, Mumbai	Karayil *et al*, 1998
	Six honeys from the West Indies of unspecified floral origin	James *et al*, 1972
	Buckwheat, tarweed, manuka, *Melaleuca* and saw palmetto honeys	Mundo *et al*, 2004
Pseudomonas aeruginosa	Unspecified, various honeys from Oman, Uganda, Tanzania, Nigeria and South Africa	Al-Jabri *et al*, 2003
	Leptospermum scoparium, Pasture honey, New Zealand	Cooper *et al*, 2002a
	Syzygium cumini, India	Subrahmanyam *et al*, 2001
	Unspecified type and number of Egyptian honeys	Zaghloul *et al*, 2001
	Lime, Acacia and fruit tree honey, country unspecified, possibly the Netherlands	Postmes *et al*, 1993
	Leptospermum scoparium, Knightia excelsa, New Zealand	Willix *et al*, 1992
	Unspecified, Saudi Arabia	Ali *et al*, 1991
	15 unprocessed honey samples of unspecified floral origin from Sudan	Farouk *et al*, 1988

Table 3.1: *Cont*

Pseudomonas aeruginosa cont	Unspecified, South Africa	Jeddar *et al*, 1985
	An unspecified number of honeys from Nigeria, one English, and one German honey were used to prepare honey distillates	Obaseiki-Ebor *et al*, 1983
	Unspecified	Ott and Morris, 2008
	31 honeys, including some of Spanish origin	Gallardo-Chacon *et al*, 2008
	Algerian honeys, including thistle, multifloral, *Eucalyptus*, orange and jujube	Boukraa *et al*, 2008a
	Eucalyptus, lavender and chestnut honeys	Wojtyczka *et al*, 2007
	Melghat honey, India	Tambekar and Rathod, 2007
	Khadikraft (India), manuka (Australia), heather honey (UK)	Mullai and Menon, 2007
	Multi-floral Turkish honeys from different regions	Mercan *et al*, 2007
	Iranian honey	Jalali *et al*, 2007
	Medihoney, a medical grade *Leptospermum* honey blend	George and Cutting, 2007
	4 Algerian, 2 Saharan honeys	Boukraa and Niar, 2007
	15 Unspecified honeys, probably Argentinean	Basualdo *et al*, 2007
	Various honeys sourced from within Venezuela	Cabrera *et al*, 2006
	Lavender, manuka, paterson's curse, red stringy bark, rewa rewa, rosemary and Medihoney, a medical grade *Leptospermum* honey blend	Wilkinson and Cavanagh, 2005
	25 Costa Rican honeys	Estrada *et al*, 2005
	Ethiopian honeys	Andargachew *et al*, 2004
Salmonella spp.	Trefoil, Egypt	Wahdan, 1998
	Langnese, Germany	El-Sukhon *et al*, 1994
	Unspecified, South Africa	Jeddar *et al*, 1985

Table 3.1: *Cont*		
Salmonella spp. cont	Cotton, clover and orange, Egypt	Radwan *et al*, 1984
	Six honeys from the West Indies of unspecified floral origin	James *et al*, 1972
	31 honeys, including some of Spanish origin	Gallardo-Chacon *et al*, 2008
	25 Costa Rican honeys	Estrada *et al*, 2005
	Nigerian honey	Adebolu, 2005
	Buckwheat, tarweed, manuka, *Melaleuca* and saw palmetto honeys	Mundo *et al*, 2004
Salmonella typhi	Unspecified, Nigeria	Obi *et al*, 1994
	Melghat honey, India	Tambekar and Rathod, 2007
	Ethiopian honeys	Andargachew *et al*, 2004
Salmonella typhimurium	Unprocessed buckwheat and blueberry, processed safflower, avocado and clover honeys	Taormina *et al*, 2001
	Knightia excelsa, Leptospermum scoparium, New Zealand	Willix *et al*, 1992
	Melghat honey, India	Tambekar and Rathod, 2007
	20 honeys from the Czech Republic	Vorlova *et al*, 2005
	Saudi Arabian honeys	Al-Hindi, 2005
Serratia marcescens	*Knightia excelsa, Leptospermum scoparium,* New Zealand	Willix *et al*, 1992
	Unspecified, South Africa	Jeddar *et al*, 1985
	An unspecified number of honeys from Nigeria, one English, and one German honey were used to prepare honey distillates	Obaseiki-Ebor *et al*, 1983
	Six honeys from the West Indies of unspecified floral origin	James *et al*, 1972
Shigella spp.	Trefoil, Egypt	Wahdan, 1998
	Six honeys from the West Indies of unspecified floral origin	James *et al*, 1972

Table 3.1: *Cont*		
Shigella spp. cont	Ethiopian honeys	Andargachew *et al*, 2004
Shigella boydii	Unspecified, Nigeria	Obi *et al*, 1994
	Unspecified, South Africa	Jeddar *et al*, 1985
Shigella dysenteriae	Langnese, Germany	El-Sukhon *et al*, 1994
	Nigerian honey	Adebolu, 2005
Shigella flexneri	Artisan orange, industrial orange and artisan citrus honey, Italy	Sinigaglia *et al*, 2000
Shigella sonnei	Unprocessed buckwheat and blueberry, processed safflower, avocado and clover honeys	Taormina *et al*, 2001
	31 honeys, including some of Spanish origin	Gallardo-Chacon *et al*, 2008
Staphylococcus spp.	Six honeys from the West Indies of unspecified floral origin	James *et al*, 1972
	15 Unspecified honeys, probably Argentinean	Basualdo *et al*, 2007
Staphylococcus aureus	Unspecified, various honeys from Oman, Uganda, Tanzania, Nigeria and South Africa	Al-Jabri *et al*, 2003
	Unspecified type and number of Egyptian honeys	Zaghloul *et al*, 2001
	Leptospermum scoparium, Knightia excelsa, New Zealand	Allen and Molan, 1997
	Langnese, Germany	El-Sukhon *et al*, 1994
	Lime, Acacia and fruit tree honey, country unspecified, possibly the Netherlands	Postmes *et al*, 1993
	Unspecified, Nigeria	Efem *et al*, 1992
	Leptospermum scoparium, Knightia excelsa, New Zealand	Willix *et al*, 1992
	Unspecified, Saudi Arabia	Ali *et al*, 1991
	Indian honeys from a variety of different floral sources and types of bees	Wakhle and Desai, 1991
	15 unprocessed honey samples of unspecified floral origin from Sudan	Farouk *et al*, 1988
	Unspecified, South Africa	Jeddar *et al*, 1985

Table 3.1: *Cont*		
Staphylococcus aureus cont	12 Swiss honeys including honeydew and chestnut, the other types were unspecified	Bogdanov, 1984
	An unspecified number of honeys from Nigeria, one English, and one German honey were used to prepare honey distillates	Obaseiki-Ebor *et al*, 1983
	Eucalyptus meullerana, E. melliodora, E. maculata, E. ochrophloia, E. albens, E. microtheca, Echium lycopsis, Australia	Wootton *et al*, 1978
	Revamil (Bfactory), a medical-grade honey of unspecified floral origin	Kwakman *et al*, 2008
	31 honeys, including some of Spanish origin	Gallardo-Chacon *et al*, 2008
	Algerian honeys, including thistle, multifloral, eucalyptus, orange and jujube	Boukraa *et al*, 2008c
	Eucalyptus cladocalyx, Leucospermum cordifolium, South African wild heather (mainly *Erica* spp.,) and *Leptospermum scoparium*	Basson and Grobler, 2008
	Eucalyptus, lavender and chestnut honeys	Wojtyczka *et al*, 2007
	Melghat honey, India	Iambekar and Rathod, 2007
	Multi-floral Turkish honeys from different regions	Mercan *et al*, 2007
	Chestnut, rhododendron and a multi-floral honey from Eastern Anatolia	Kucuk *et al*, 2007
	Iranian honey	Jalali *et al*, 2007
	15 unspecified honeys, probably Argentinean	Basualdo *et al*, 2007
	Various honeys sourced from within Lithuania	Baltrusaityte *et al*, 2007
	Various honeys sourced from within Venezuela	Cabrera *et al*, 2006
	20 honeys from the Czech Republic	Vorlova *et al*, 2005
	30 Portuguese honeys	Henriques *et al*, 2005
	25 Costa Rican honeys	Estrada *et al*, 2005

Table 3.1: *Cont*

Staphylococcus aureus cont	Acacia honey	Dugalic-Vrndic *et al*, 2005
	Honey from United Arab Emirates	Al-Waili *et al*, 2005
	Unspecified honey, mixed with beeswax and olive oil	Al-Waili, 2005
	30 honeys, Oman	Al-Jabri *et al*, 2005a; Al-Jabri *et al*, 2005b
	Saudi Arabian honeys	Al-Hindi, 2005
	Buckwheat, tarweed, manuka, *Melaleuca* and saw palmetto honeys	Mundo *et al*, 2004
	Manuka	Kouda *et al*, 2004
	Multiple non-manuka honeys from New Zealand	Brady *et al*, 2004
	Ethiopian honeys	Andargachew *et al*, 2004
	Syzygium cumini, India	Subrahmanyam *et al*, 2001
	Unprocessed buckwheat and blueberry, processed safflower, avocado and clover honeys	Taormina *et al*, 2001
	Leptospermum scoparium, pasture honey, New Zealand	Cooper *et al*, 1999
	An unspecified number of honeys from Nigeria, one English, and one German honey were used to prepare honey distillates	Obaseiki-Ebor *et al*, 1983
Staphylococcus, coagulase -	Syzygium cumini, India *Leptospermum scoparium*, pasture honey, New Zealand	Subrahmanyam *et al*, 2001 French *et al*, 2005
MRSA	*Leptospermum scoparium*, Pasture honey, New Zealand	Cooper *et al*, 2002b
	Medihoney, a medical grade *Leptospermum* honey blend	George and Cutting, 2007
Community-acquired MRSA	Heather and two other local honeys (Northern Ireland), unspecified French honey	Maeda *et al*, 2008
Staphylococcus epidermidis	Trefoil, Egypt	Wahdan, 1998
	Revamil (Bfactory), a medical-grade honey of unspecified floral origin	Kwakman *et al*, 2008

Table 3.1: *Cont*

Staphylococcus epidermidis cont	Melghat honey, India	Tambekar and Rathod, 2007
	Various honeys sourced from within Lithuania	Baltrusaityte *et al*, 2007
	15 Unspecified honeys, probably Argentinean	Basualdo *et al*, 2007
	25 Costa Rican honeys	Estrada *et al*, 2005
	10 Indian honeys	Amit *et al*, 2005
Streptococcus spp.	Lime, Acacia and fruit tree honey, country unspecified, possibly the Netherlands	Postmes *et al*, 1993
	An unspecified number of honeys from Nigeria, one English, and one German honey were used to prepare honey distillates	Obaseiki-Ebor *et al*, 1983
	Six honeys from the West Indies of unspecified floral origin	James *et al*, 1972
	31 honeys, including some of Spanish origin	Gallardo-Chacon *et al*, 2008
	Eucalyptus cladocalyx, Leucospermum cordifolium, South African wild heather (mainly *Erica* spp.), and *Leptospermum scoparium*	Basson and Grobler, 2008
	Manuka	Kouda *et al*, 2001
ß-haemolytic *Streptococcus*	Unspecified, Saudi Arabia	Ali *et al*, 1991
Streptococcus agalactiae	*Leptospermum scoparium, Knightia excelsa*, New Zealand	Allen and Molan, 1997
Streptococcus dysgalactiae	*Leptospermum scoparium, Knightia excelsa*, New Zealand	Allen and Molan, 1997
Streptococcus pyogenes	Unspecified, Nigeria	Efem *et al*, 1992
	Knightia excelsa, Leptospermum scoparium, New Zealand	Willix *et al*, 1992
	Unspecified, South Africa	Jeddar *et al*, 1985

Table 3.1: *Cont*		
Streptococcus pyogenes cont	Honey from United Arab Emirates	Al-Waili *et al*, 2005
Streptococcus pneumoniae	Trefoil, Egypt	Wahdan, 1998
Streptococcus uberis	*Leptospermum scoparium, Knightia excelsa,* New Zealand	Allen and Molan, 1997
Vibrio cholerae	Trefoil, Egypt	Wahdan, 1998
	Unspecified, Nigeria	Obi *et al*, 1994
	Unspecified, South Africa	Jeddar *et al*, 1985
Yersinia enterocolitica	Unspecified, Nigeria	Obi *et al*, 1994
Yersinia ruckeri	Trefoil, Egypt	Wahdan, 1998
Unidentified organisms from sewage, soil, tap water and air	Cotton, clover and orange, Egypt	Radwan *et al*, 1984
Unidentified organisms from air	Six honeys from the West Indies of unspecified floral origin	James *et al*, 1972

of 345 honey samples from New Zealand the antibacterial activity, expressed as the concentration of a standard antiseptic, phenol, ranged from the equivalent of less than 2%, w/v, phenol to 58%, w/v, phenol, with a median of 13.6 (Allen *et al,* 1991). Similarly, in a survey of over 500 Australian honeys the antibacterial activity ranged from undetectable to 34% phenol equivalence, with a mean of around 13% for all of the honeys tested, and a mean of around 17% for all of the honeys with detectable activity (Irish, University of Sydney, personal communication). Variations in activity have also been found in Portuguese (Henriques *et al*, 2005) and Welsh honeys (Cooper *et al*, in press).

If honey is to be used as a therapeutic agent in modern medicine, choosing the correct type is crucial for optimal outcomes. It is important to know that there can also be a great deal of variation between the activity levels of different samples of the same types of honey. For example, not all *Leptospermum* honeys produced in New Zealand exhibit significant non-peroxide levels of activity (Allen *et al,* 1991; Stephens *et al,* 2005); there are over 80 different *Leptospermum* species in Australia, but only a few of these produce honeys with exceptional activity (Irish, University of Sydney, personal communication). In addition, the way the honey is harvested, processed and packaged should be strictly controlled, as is discussed in *Chapter 5*.

Honey-based wound care products have been registered with the medical regulatory authorities as wound care agents in Australia, Canada, the European Union, Hong Kong, New Zealand and the USA. In many instances, they use manuka honey from New Zealand or the equivalent honey produced from other *Leptospermum* species in Australia, but buckwheat, multifloral and honeys of unspecified floral origin are also used. The simplest way of ensuring that the most beneficial type of honey is employed as a wound dressing is to use one that is appropriately registered as a medical product, rather than as a food product. However, as summarised in *Table 3.1*, there are numerous honeys from around the world that exhibit significant levels of antibacterial activity. Many of these could be employed as infection control agents, especially in emergency situations such as natural disasters, including tsunamis, earthquakes and cyclones. These phenomena leave countless people injured and at risk of life-threatening infections from wounds that they have sustained, often with little access to immediate medical care.

The potent antibacterial activity of Leptospermum honey

The potent, non-hydrogen peroxide dependent antibacterial activity found in *Leptospermum scoparium* (manuka) honey from New Zealand was first identified by Peter Molan (Molan and Russell, 1988). Since then, there have been numerous investigations using this honey. The activity of this honey is particularly important because it is heat stable and it is not reduced in the presence of catalase, which is found in wound tissues.

Some examples of investigations using *Leptospermum* honey (manuka from New Zealand) with defined levels of activity, and where standardised methods were employed are summarised in *Table 3.2*. These studies have tested the honey-susceptibility of problematic wound pathogens, including those with innate or acquired antibiotic-resistance. Similar results were reported with an Australian active *Leptospermum* medical grade honey blend (George and Cutting, 2007). In the study, a broad range of antibiotic-resistant bacteria were tested including *Staphylococcus aureus* (including MRSA), vancomycin-resistant *Enterococcus* (VRE), *Acinetobacter baumannii*, *P. aeruginosa* and extended spectrum beta-lactamase (ESBL) producing isolates of *Escherichia coli* and *Klebsiella pneumoniae*. We have also found similar results using medical grade *Leptospermum* honeys against multiple clinical isolates of *S. aureus* (including MRSA), multi drug-resistant members of the Enterobacteriaceae family (such as *Citrobacter*, *Enterobacteria*, *Escherichia*, *Klebsiella*, *Morganella* and *Serratia*) and *Acinetobacter* (Blair *et al*, manuscript in preparation).

Of the many investigations into the antibacterial activity of honey, only a relatively few have been performed on facultative organisms growing in the absence of oxygen or on strict anaerobes (Efem *et al*, 1992; Postmes *et al*, 1993). However, although probably underreported in clinical microbiology, anaerobically growing pathogens often have significant detrimental effects in both colonised and infected wounds (Howell-Jones *et al*, 2005). The *in vitro* activity of antibiotics is most often studied under aerobic conditions. However, it is possible that certain drugs have different efficacies under aerobic and anaerobic conditions. For example, when the efficacies of five fluoroquinolones against *S. aureus* were

Table 3.2: Laboratory testing of manuka honey using clinical isolates

Organisms tested	Number of cultures	Non-peroxide phenol equivalent %, w/v	Mean honey MIC % v/v	Range of honey MIC values % v/v	References
Burkholderia cepacia	20	13.2	2.9	2.1–5.0	Cooper et al, 2000
Coagulase-negative staphylococci	18	16.8	3.4	3.0–4.0	French et al, 2005
P. aeruginosa	17	18.0	7.49	4.0–9.0	Cooper et al, 2002a
S. aureus, MSSA	58	14.8	2.88	2.0–3.0	Cooper et al, 1999
S. aureus, MRSA	18	18.0	2.98	2.7–3.0	Cooper et al, 2002b
Vancomycin-sensitive enterococci	7	18.0	4.92	4.66–5.0	Cooper et al, 2002b
Vancomycin-resistant enterococci	20	18.0	4.61	3.83–5.0	Cooper et al, 2002b

investigated under both aerobic and anaerobic conditions, all of the antibiotics had a delayed bactericidal effect in the absence of oxygen (Zabinski *et al*, 1995). Work from our laboratory shows that selected medical grade honeys, particularly *Leptospermum* ones from Australia and New Zealand, discussed below, are effective against strict anaerobes such as *Clostridium* spp., as well as facultative organisms grown in the presence or absence of oxygen. The honeys also had clinically achievable MICs against antibiotic-resistant anaerobes (Blair *et al*, unpublished work).

Infections caused by pathogens such as MRSA, *P. aeruginosa* and antibiotic-resistant members of the Enterobacteriaceae family are alarmingly common. Those caused by opportunistic pathogens such as *Burkholderia cepacia* and *Acinetobacter* spp. occur less frequently, although the incidences of these are increasing. However, regardless of their frequency, the problem of antibiotic-resistance makes all of their infections more difficult and expensive to treat. Despite this, all of these organisms are susceptible to the antibacterial activity of *Leptospermum* honey, even when it is significantly diluted.

The low MICs of this honey are crucial because they demonstrate that selected *Leptospermum* honeys can maintain significant levels of antibacterial activity, even in heavily exudating wounds. These honeys could be diluted up to 20 times in the wound bed and still be effective against any microbes present, which is an important clinical consideration. Furthermore, the broad-spectrum activity of honey, along with its efficacy against antibiotic-resistant pathogens, means that neither the identity nor drug-susceptibility profile of an infective agent needs to be elucidated before effective treatment can commence. This is in stark contrast to antibiotic drug treatment. The use of broad-spectrum drugs adds to the pressures that have been associated with the emergence of resistant organisms, and can have wider effects on the normal flora of the patient. However, from the physician's and the patient's point of view, it is not usually an option to wait for identification and susceptibility information before beginning treatment. Thus, there is a conflict between the good of individual patients (who may benefit from immediate broad-spectrum antibiotic treatment) and the good of society as a whole (which would benefit from a reduced use of antibiotics, especially broad-spectrum ones). If there were a greater use of honey, such as medicinal grade *Leptospermum*, in areas such as wound care, patients would benefit without producing a negative effect on society as a whole.

Effectiveness against non-bacterial pathogens

Although it will not be discussed in detail here, honey also shows antifungal activity against the pathogenic yeasts such as *Candida* spp. (Obaseiki-Ebor *et al*, 1983; Efem *et al*, 1992; Adeleye and Opiah, 2003; Al-Waili *et al*, 2005; Irish *et al*, 2006; Boukraa *et al*, 2008b) and filamentous fungal pathogens including dermatophytes (Efem *et al*, 1992; Brady *et al*, 1996; Al-Waili, 2004a), and *Aspergillus* spp. (Efem *et al*, 1992; Wellford *et al*, 1978; Boukraa and Bouchegrane, 2007, as well as antiviral properties (Zeina *et al*, 1996; Al-Waili, 2004b), antiprotozoal activity (Zeina *et al*, 1997), and antihelminth actions (Kilicoglu *et al*, 2006).

Conclusion

Although honey is not a uniform product, its major constituents combine to make conditions unsuitable for the growth of a wide range of microbial species. Laboratory tests confirm it possesses a broad spectrum of antimicrobial activity. Even after dilution by body fluids, honeys with the ability to generate hydrogen peroxide and those that contain additional phytochemical antimicrobial components have the potential to be effective antimicrobial agents *in vivo*. The benefits of honey in inhibiting wound-associated organisms will be explored in the next chapter.

References

Adams CJ, Boult CH, Deadman BJ, *et al* (2008) Isolation by HPLC and characterisation of the bioactive fraction of New Zealand manuka (*Leptospermum scoparium*) honey. *Carbohydrate Res* **343**: 651–9

Adebolu TT (2005) Effect of natural honey on local isolates of diarrhea-causing bacteria in southwestern Nigeria. *Afr J Biotechnol* **4**: 1172–4

Adeleye IA, Opiah L (2003) Antimicrobial activity of extracts of local cough mixtures on upper respiratory tract bacterial pathogens. *West Ind Med J* **52**: 188–90

Al-Hindi RR (2005) The inhibitory activity of honey and 'honey pastes' against selected foodborne bacterial pathogens. *Arab Universities J Agricultural Sci* **13**: 807–13

Al-Jabri AA, Nzeako B, Al Mahrooqi Z, Al Naqdy A, Nsanze H (2003) *In vitro* antibacterial activity of Omani and African honey. *Br J Biomed Sci* **60**: 1–4

Al-Jabri AA, Al Hosni SA, Nzeako B, Nsanze H (2005a) Antistaphylococcal activity of Omani honey in combination with bovine milk. *Br J Biomed Sci* **62**: 92–3

Al-Jabri AA, Al-Hosni SA, Nzeako BC, Al-Mahrooqi ZH, Nsanze H (2005b) Antibacterial activity of Omani honey alone and in combination with gentamicin. *Saudi Med J* **26**: 767–71

Al-Somal NA, Coley KE, Molan PC, Hancock BM (1994) Susceptibility of *Helicobacter pylori* to the antibacterial activity of manuka honey. *J Roy Soc Med* **87**: 9—12

Al-Waili NS (2004a) An alternative treatment for pityriasis versicolor, tinea cruris, tinea corporis and tinea faciei with topical application of honey, olive oil and beeswax mixture: an open pilot study. *Complement Ther Med* **12**: 45–7

Al-Waili NS (2004b) Topical honey application vs. acyclovir for the treatment of recurrent herpes simplex lesions. *Med Sci Monitor* **10**: MT94–MT98

Al-Waili NS (2005) Mixture of honey, beeswax and olive oil inhibits growth of *Staphylococcus aureus* and *Candida albicans*. *Arch Med Res* **36**: 10–13

Al-Waili NS, Akmal M, Al-Waili F, Saloom KY, Ali A (2005) The antimicrobial potential of honey from United Arab Emirates on some microbial isolates. *Med Sci Monitor* **11**: BR433–BR438

Ali AT, Chowdhury MN, al Humayyd MS (1991) Inhibitory effect of natural honey on *Helicobacter pylori*. *Trop Gastroenterol* **12**: 139–43

Allen KL, Molan PC, Reid GM (1991) A survey of the antibacterial activity of some New Zealand honeys. *J Pharm Pharmacol* **43**: 817–22

Allen KL, Molan PC (1997) The sensitivity of mastitis-causing bacteria to the antibacterial activity of honey. *N Z J Agricultural Resh* **40**: 537–40

Amit K, Richa K, Anjana K, Kashyap MK (2005) Indian honey: a natural product with antibacterial activity against antibiotic resistant pathogens, an *in vitro* study. *Pakistan J Biol Sci* **8**: 190–3

Andargachew M, Belay T, Fetene D (2004) *In vitro* assessment of the antimicrobial potential of honey on common human pathogens. *Ethiopian J Health Development* **18**: 107–11

Baltrusaityte V, Venskutonis PR, Ceksteryte V (2007) Antibacterial activity of honey and beebread of different origin against *S. aureus* and *S. epidermidis*. *Food Technol Biotechnol* **45**: 201–8

Basson NJ, Grobler SR (2008) Antimicrobial activity of two South African honeys produced from indigenous *Leucospermum cordifolium* and Erica species on selected micro-organisms. *BMC Complement Altern Med* **8**: 41

Basualdo C, Sgroy V, Finola MS, Marioli JM (2007) Comparison of the antibacterial activity of honey from different provenance against bacteria usually isolated from skin wounds. *Vet Microbiol* **124**: 375–81

Bogdanov S (1984) Characterization of antibacterial substances in honey. *Lebensmittel-Wissenschaft Technologie* **17**: 74–6

Boukraa L, Bouchegrane S (2007) Additive action of honey and starch against *Candida albicans* and *Aspergillus niger*. *Revista Iberoamericana de Micologia* 24: 309–11

Boukraa L, Niar A (2007) Sahara honey shows higher potency against *Pseudomonas aeruginosa* compared to North Algerian types of honey. *J Medicinal Food* 10: 712–4

Boukraa L, Benbarek H, Aissat S (2008a) Synergistic action of starch and honey against *Pseudomonas aeruginosa* in correlation with diastase number. *J Altern Complement Med* 14: 181–4

Boukraa L, Benbarek H, Moussa A (2008b) Synergistic action of starch and honey against *Candida albicans* in correlation with diastase number. *Braz J Microbiol* 39: 40–3

Boukraa L, Niar A, Benbarek H, Benhanifia M (2008c) Additive action of royal jelly and honey against *Staphylococcus aureus*. *J Medicinal Food* 11: 190–2

Brady N, Molan P, Bang L (2004) A survey of non-manuka New Zealand honeys for antibacterial and antifungal activities. *J Apic Res* 43: 47–52

Brady NF, Molan PC, Harfoot CG (1996) The sensitivity of dermatophytes to the antimicrobial activity of manuka honey and other honey. *Pharm Sci* 2: 471–3

Brudzynski K (2006) Effect of hydrogen peroxide on antibacterial activities of Canadian honeys. *Can J Microbiol* 52: 1228–37

Cabrera L, Cespedes E, Nava R, de Rodriguez GO (2006) Non-peroxide antibacterial activity in Zulia honeys. *Revista Cientifica-Facultad De Ciencias Veterinarias* 16: 556–63

Cooper R, Molan P (1999) The use of honey as an antiseptic in managing *Pseudomonas* infection. *J Wound Care* 8: 161–4

Cooper RA, Molan PC, Harding KG (1999) Antibacterial activity of honey against strains of *Staphylococcus aureus* from infected wounds. *J Roy Soc Med* 92: 283–5

Cooper RA, Wigley P, Burton NF (2000) Susceptibility of multiresistant strains of *Burkholderia cepacia* to honey. *Letters Appl Microbiol* 31: 20–4

Cooper RA, Halas E, Molan PC (2002a) The efficacy of honey in inhibiting strains of *Pseudomonas aeruginosa* from infected burns. *J Burn Care Rehabil* 23: 366–70

Cooper RA, Molan PC, Harding KG (2002b) The sensitivity to honey of Gram-positive cocci of clinical significance isolated from wounds. *J Appl Microbiol* 93: 857–63

Cooper RA, Wheat E-J, Burton NF (in press) Wound healing characteristics of Welsh honeys. *J Apicul Res*

Curda L, Plockova M (1995) Impedance measurement of growth of lactic-acid bacteria in dairy cultures with honey addition. *Int Dairy J* 5: 727–33

DeMera JH, Angert ER (2004) Comparison of the antimicrobial activity of honey produced by *Tetragonisca angustula* (*Meliponinae*) and *Apis mellifera* from different phytogeographic regions of Costa Rica. *Apidologie* 35: 411–7

Dugalic-Vrndic N, Pesic-Mikulec D, Baltic M (2005) Acacia honey from different localities and its effect on _Staphylococcus aureus_ and Listeria monocytogenes. _Veterinarski Glasnik_ 59: 283–7

Efem SEE, Udoh KT, Iwara CI (1992) The antimicrobial spectrum of honey and its clinical significance. _Infection_ 20: 227–9

Elbagoury EFA, Rasmy S (1993) Antibacterial action of natural honey on anaerobic _Bacteroides. Egyptian Dent J_ 39: 381–6

El-Kamali HH (2000) Folk medicinal use of some animal products in Central Sudan. _J Ethnopharmacol_ 72: 279–82

El-Sukhon SN, Abuharfeil N, Sallal AK (1994) Effect of honey on bacterial growth and spore germination. _J Food Protection_ 57: 918–20

Estrada H, Gamboa MD, Chaves C, Arias ML (2005) Evaluation of the antimicrobial action of honey against _Staphylococcus aureus, Staphylococcus epidermidis, Pseudomonas aeruginosa, Escherichia coli, Salmonella enteritidis, Listeria monocytogenes_ and _Aspergillus niger_. Evaluation of its microbiological charge. _Archivos Latinoamericanos De Nutricion_ 55: 167–71

Fangio MF, Iurlina MO, Fritz R (2007) Antimicrobial activity of honey against _Escherichia coli. Revista Argentina de Microbiologia_ 39: 120–3

Farouk A, Hassan T, Kashif H, Khalid SA, Mutawali I, Wadi M (1988) Studies on Sudanese bee honey laboratory and clinical evaluation. _Int J Crude Drug Res_ 26: 161–8

French VM, Cooper RA, Molan PC (2005) The antibacterial activity of honey against coagulase-negative staphylococci. _J Antimicrob Chemother_ 56: 228–31

Gallardo-Chacon JJ, Casellies M, Izquierdo-Pulido M, Rius N (2008) Inhibitory activity of monofloral and multifloral honeys against bacterial pathogens. J _Apic Res_ 47: 131–6

Garedew A, Schmolz E, Lamprecht I (2003) The antimicrobial activity of honey of the stingless bee _Trigona_ spp. _J Apic Sci_ 47: 37–49

George NM, Cutting KF (2007) Antibacterial honey (Medihoney™): _in-vitro_ activity against clinical isolates of MRSA, VRE, and other multiresistant gram-negative organisms including _Pseudomonas aeruginosa. Wounds — A Compendium of Clinical Research and Practice_ 19: 231–6

Henriques A, Burton NF, Cooper RA (2005) Antibacterial activity of selected Portuguese honeys. _J Apic Res_ 44: 119–23

Irish J, Carter DA, Shokohi T, Blair SE (2006) Honey has an antifungal effect against _Candida_ species. _Med Mycol_ 44: 289–91

Irish J, Carter DA, Blair SE, Heard TA (2008) Antibacterial activity of honey from the Australian stingless bee _Trigona carbonaria. Int J Antimicrob Agents_ 32: 89–90

Jalali FSS, Ehsani A, Tajik H, Ashtari S (2007) _In vitro_ assessment of efficacy of gamma irradiation on the antimicrobial activity of Iranian honey. _J Animal Veterinary Advances_ 6: 996–9

James OBO, Segree W, Ventura AK (1972) Some antibacterial properties of Jamaican honey. *West Indian Med J* **21**: 7–17

Jeddar A, Kharsany A, Ramsaroop UG, Bhamjee A, Haffejee, IE, Moosa A (1985) The antibacterial action of honey — an *in vitro* study. *South Afr Med J* **67**: 257–8

Karayil S, Deshpande SD, Koppikar GV (1998) Effect of honey on multidrug resistant organisms and its synergistic action with three common antibiotics. *J Postgrad Med* **44**: 93–6

Kilicoglu B, Kismet K, Koru O, Tanyuksel M, Oruc MT, Sorkun K, Ali Akkus M (2006) The scolicidal effects of honey. *Adv Ther* **23**(6): 1085–91

Kouda M, Homma S, Syu E, Samejima K, Nakayama M (2004) Antibacterial activity of green tea extract, manuka honey and *Melaleuca alternifolia* against clinical isolated organisms. *Aroma Res* **5**: 364–70

Kucuk M, Kolayli S, Karaoglu S, Ulusoy E, Baltaci C, Candan F (2007) Biological activities and chemical composition of three honeys of different types from Anatolia. *Food Chemistry* **100**: 526–34

Kwakman PHS, Van den Akker JPC, Guclu A, *et al* (2008) Medical-grade honey kills antibiotic-resistant bacteria *in vitro* and eradicates skin colonization. *Clin Infect Dis* **46**: 1677–82

Maeda Y, Loughrey A, Earle JA, Millar BC, Rao JR, Kearns A, *et al* (2008) Antibacterial activity of honey against community-associated methicillin-resistant *Staphylococcus aureus* (CA-MRSA). *Complement Ther Clin Pract* **14**(2): 77–82

Martins SCS, Albuquerque LMB, Matos JHG, Silva GC, Pereira AIB (1997) Antibacterial activity of honeys of Africanized honey bees (*Apis mellifera*) and native bees (*Melipona scutellaris, M. subnitida and Scaptotrigona bipunctata*) in the state of Ceara. *Higiene Alimentar* **11**: 50–3

Mercan N, Guvensenz A, Celik A, Katircioglu H (2007) Antimicrobial activity and pollen composition of honey samples collected from different provinces in Turkey. *Natural Product Res* **21**: 187–95

Miorin PL, Junior NCL, Custodio AR, Bretz WA, Marcucci MC (2003) Antibacterial activity of honey and propolis from *Apis mellifera* and *Tetragonisca angustula* against *Staphylococcus aureus*. *J Appl Microbiol* **95**: 913–20

Molan PC (1992) The antibacterial nature of honey: 1. The nature of the antibacterial activity. *Bee World* **73**(1): 5–28

Molan PC, Russell KM (1988) Non-peroxide antibacterial activity in some New Zealand honeys. *J Apic Res* **27**: 62–7

Mullai V, Menon T (2007) Bactericidal activity of different types of honey against clinical and environmental isolates of *Pseudomonas aeruginosa*. *J Altern Complement Med* **13**: 439–41

Mundo MA, Padilla-Zakour OI, Worobo RW (2004) Growth inhibition of foodborne pathogens and food spoilage organisms by select raw honeys. *Int J Food Microbiol* **97**: 1–8

Obaseiki-Ebor EE, Afonya TCA, Onyekweli AO (1983) Preliminary report on the antimicrobial activity of honey distillate. _J Pharm Pharmacol_ **35**: 748–9

Obi CL, Ugoji EO, Edun SA, Lawal SF, Anyiwo CE (1994) The antibacterial effect of honey on diarrhoea causing bacterial agents isolated in Lagos, Nigeria. _Afr J Med Med Sci_ **23**: 257–60

Osato MS, Reddy SG, Graham DY (1999) Osmotic effect of honey on growth and viability of _Helicobacter pylori_. _Dig Dis Sci_ **44**: 462–4

Ott JA, Morris AN (2008) Homeopathic alternatives to conventional antibiotics. _Bios_ **79**: 50–5

Postmes T, Vandenbogaard AE, Hazen M (1993) Honey for wounds, ulcers, and skin graft preservation. _Lancet_ **341**: 756–7

Radwan SS, El-Essawy AA, Sarhan MM (1984) Experimental evidence for the occurrence in honey of specific substances sctive against microorganisms. _Zentralblatt Fur Mikrobiologie_ **139**: 249–55

Shamala TR, Jyothi YPS, Saibaba P (2002) Antibacterial effect of honey on the _in vitro_ and _in vivo_ growth of _Escherichia coli_. _World J Microbiol Biotechnol_ **18**: 863–5

Sinigaglia M, Corbo MR, Massa S (2000) Effect of three honey types on _Escherichia coli_ O157:H7 and _Shigella flexneri_. _Adv Food Sci_ **22**: 156–60

Stephens JMC, Molan PC, Clarkson BD (2005). A review of _Leptospermum scoparium_ (_Myrtaceae_) in New Zealand. _N Z J Botany_ **43**: 431–49

Subrahmanyam M, Archan H, Pawar SG (2001) Antibacterial activity of honey on bacteria isolated from wounds. _Ann Burns Fire Disasters_ **14**: 22–4

Tambekar DH, Rathod GN (2007) Indian melghat honey: a prospective antibiotic. _J Pharmacol Toxicol_ **2**: 80–4

Taormina PJ, Niemira BA, Beuchat LR (2001) Inhibitory activity of honey against foodborne pathogens as influenced by the presence of hydrogen peroxide and level of antioxidant power. _Int J Food Microbiol_ **69**: 217–25

Torres A, Garedew A, Schmolz E, Lamprecht I (2004) Calorimetric investigation of the antimicrobial action and insight into the chemical properties of 'angelita' honey — a product of the stingless bee _Tetragonisca angustula_ from Colombia. _Thermochimica Acta_ **415**: 107–13

Vorlova L, Karpiskova R, Chabiniokova I, Kalabova K, Brazdova Z (2005) The antimicrobial activity of honeys produced in the Czech Republic. _Czech J Animal Sci_ **50**: 376–84

Wahdan HAL (1998) Causes of the antimicrobial activity of honey. _Infection_ **26**: 26–31

Wakhle DM, Desai DB (1991) Estimation of antibacterial activity of some Indian honeys. _Ind Bee J_ **53**: 80–90

Wellford TET, Eadie T, Llewellyn GC (1978) Evaluating inhibitory action of honey on fungal growth, sporulation, and aflatoxin production. _Zeitschrift Fur Lebensmittel-Untersuchung Und-Forschung_ **166**: 280–3

Wilkinson JM, Cavanagh HMA (2005) Antibacterial activity of 13 honeys against _Escherichia coli_ and _Pseudomonas aeruginosa_. _J Medicinal Food_ **8**: 100–3

Willix DJ, Molan PC, Harfoot CG (1992) A comparison of the sensitivity of wound infecting species of bacteria to the antibacterial activity of manuka honey and other honey. *J Appl Bacteriol* **73**: 388–94

Wojtyczka RD, Kabala-Dzik A, Stojko J, Kepa M, Idzik D, Stojko R, *et al* (2007) Antimicrobial activity analysis a different kinds of honey. *Zywienie Czlowieka i Metabolizm* **34**: 1322–6

Wootton M, Edwards RA, Rowse A (1978) Antibacterial properties of some Australian honeys. *Food Tech Aust* **30**: 175–6

Zaghloul AA, El-Shattawy HH, Kassem AA, Ibrahim EA, Reddy IK, Khan MA (2001) Honey, a prospective antibiotic: extraction, formulation, and stability. *Pharmazie* **56**: 643–7

Zeina B, Othman O, al-Assad S (1996) Effect of honey versus thyme on Rubella virus survival *in vitro*. *J Altern Complement Med* **2**: 345–8

Zeina B, Alassad S, Zohra BI (1997) The effects of honey on leishmania parasites: An *in vitro* study. *Tropical Doctor* **27**: 36–8

Chapter 4

Challenges in Modern Wound Microbiology and the Role for Honey

Rose Cooper and Shona Blair

The greatest potential medical use of topical honey in modern medicine is in the control of microorganisms in wounds, particularly for infection control. Patients who acquire nosocomial wound infections have significantly higher mortality rates than those that do not (Paul *et al*, 2007; Young *et al*, 2008). Surgical site infections, which remain a source of postoperative morbidity, are the most common nosocomial infections in patients undergoing surgery (Filius and Gyssens, 2002; Yasunaga *et al*, 2007). Infections in burns units are also common, reported in up to 55% of admissions (Appelgren *et al*, 2002; Santucci *et al*, 2003; Silla *et al*, 2006; Wibbenmeyer *et al*, 2006), where they jeopardise the success of grafts and also cause over 50% of burn victim deaths (Albrecht *et al*, 2006; Church *et al*, 2006). Predictably, nosocomial infections also lead to significantly higher healthcare costs (Stone *et al*, 2005; Yasunaga *et al*, 2007). To compound these issues, the appearance of antimicrobial resistance in bacteria is a problem of growing significance in dermatological and surgical wound infections (Filius and Gyssens, 2002). However, despite the introduction of numerous control measures around the world, the problems caused by antibiotic-resistant organisms are increasing and unless new antimicrobials are found the field of wound management will lose much of the ground it has gained in the twentieth century. The development of a new antimicrobial has been estimated to cost US$400–800 million, and there are a decreasing number of these drugs in the pipeline. Most alarmingly, current antimicrobial drug development is insufficient to meet society's needs (Spellberg *et al*, 2004).

Here we highlight *Staphylococcus aureus* as an example of an extremely problematic antibiotic-resistant wound pathogen.

This aggressive pathogen has become increasingly resistant to antibiotics, narrowing the choice of useful agents, and placing a huge burden on healthcare systems around the world. Skin and soft tissue infections caused by methicillin-resistant *S. aureus* (MRSA) are among the most common that occur, and they are linked to lengthened wound healing times, an increase in adverse postoperative outcomes and increased mortality (Chung *et al*, 2008; Edris and Reed, 2008; Kennedy *et al*, 2008; Klevens *et al*, 2007; Kuehnert *et al*, 2005). Nosocomial MRSA infection is associated with higher morbidity, mortality and medical costs than infection caused by methicillin-susceptible *S. aureus* (Cosgrove *et al*, 2003; Engemann *et al*, 2003). Community-acquired MRSA (CA-MRSA) is now a common cause of disease in both children and adults (Avdic and Cosgrove, 2008). Most (>90%) CA-MRSA infections present as minor skin and soft tissue infections (Popovich and Hota, 2008; Stryjewski and Chambers, 2008), although the infections may also be severe and invasive, such as necrotising fasciitis (Miller *et al*, 2005). In addition, MRSA is often resistant to other treatments such as ciprofloxacin, clindamycin, daptomycin, fusidic acid, linezolid, mupirocin, rifampin, tetracycline and vancomycin (Popovich and Hota, 2008). Innovative therapeutic approaches to the management of these infections are urgently needed.

Despite being a remarkably osmotolerant organism that can survive on intact skin and surfaces, *S. aureus* is extremely sensitive to the antibacterial activity of certain honeys, such as active *Leptospermum* honeys from New Zealand and Australia (Cooper *et al*, 1999; Cooper *et al*, 2002b; French *et al*, 2005; George and Cutting, 2007; Lusby *et al*, 2005). Most importantly, this honey has been shown to be just as effective against multiple drug-resistant strains as it is against drug-sensitive strains. This is the case not only with *S. aureus* (including MRSA) but also with numerous other Gram-positive and Gram-negative pathogens (Cooper *et al*, 2000; Cooper *et al*, 2002a; Cooper *et al*, 2002b; French *et al*, 2005; Blair *et al*, unpublished work).

Using honey to control pathogens in wounds

It is important to remember that laboratory tests only provide an indication of the relative sensitivities of test organisms to honey samples and that clinical efficacy is determined by *in vivo* observations.

There are many publications within the medical literature that describe the clearance of infection following the topical application of honey (reviewed in Molan, 2006). More recently, the number of instances where the eradication of an antibiotic-resistant bacterium (MRSA) from wounds has been described has increased. Examples include: a colonised, hydroxyurea-induced leg ulcer (Natarajan et al, 2001); chronic leg ulcers (Dunford et al, 2001; Chambers, 2006; Gethin and Cowman, 2008); a diabetic foot ulcer in a patient facing amputation (Eddy and Gideonsen, 2005); chronic wounds in maxofacial surgery patients (Visavedia et al, 2008) and wounds in children undergoing treatment for cancers (Simon et al 2006; Blaser et al, 2007). In most of these cases attempts to control MRSA with systemic antibiotics and antiseptics had failed. These cases illustrate the potential of honey to prevent and clear infection, and to reduce the risk of cross-infection. Additionally, inhibition of antibiotic-resistant bacteria in in vitro tests and eradication from healthy colonised skin by a medical grade honey produced under controlled conditions in the Netherlands has been described (Kwakman et al, 2008).

Another benefit to using honey in wounds is its ability to remove malodour. The involvement of anaerobic and facultative bacteria in the production of offensive smell was established by comparing odour severity with microbial flora in infected and non-infected leg ulcers (Bowler et al, 1999). The removal of malodour following the use of honey has been reported in leg ulcers (Gethin and Cowman, 2005; Dunford and Hanano, 2004) and pressure ulcers (van der Weyden, 2003). This could be due to the inhibition of anaerobic bacteria (_Chapter 3_), or to a metabolic effect of honey as discussed in _Chapter 2_.

Antimicrobial interventions in wounds

Skin is normally disinfected before elective wounding, but other than immediately after disinfection, the presence of microorganisms as mixed communities in wounds is not considered to be unusual (Bowler et al, 2001). Despite extensive research the influence of microorganisms on the pathophysiology of wounds is not fully understood. Multiple interactions impact on healing and boundaries between microbial and host factors are hard to delineate (Vowden et al 2008). Additionally, inflammation is caused by the initial wounding event, as well as the development of infection (Edwards and Harding

2004; Jones *et al*, 2004). Acute infections always interrupt the normal healing process (Bucknell, 1980; Robson *et al*, 1990) and must be controlled, yet it is not essential to sterilise a wound to promote healing. The pathogens commonly associated with wound infection are staphylococci, streptococci, pseudomonads and anaerobes. In part, modern management approaches have been influenced by a study in which the effect of topical agents, by decreasing bacterial load in infected ulcers, was shown to improve healing rates (Lyman *et al*, 1970). Antimicrobial interventions cannot be justified on this premise alone and are not necessarily effective on persistent infections. Antibiotics should be reserved for acute infections and targeted at specific pathogens (Eron *et al* 2003). Judicious use should also be made of topical agents, as resistance to antiseptics has been found (McDonnell and Russell, 1999).

Chronic wounds and bacteria

Chronic wounds represent an enormous burden to modern medical practice. In the UK it has been estimated that approximately 3% of the total National Health Service expenditure (£2.3–3.1 billion during 2005–2006) was utilised on 200,000 patients with chronic wounds (such as venous leg ulcers, pressure ulcers or foot ulcers) (Posnett and Franks, 2008). In an ageing population, with increasing prevalence of diabetes and obesity, the number of chronic wounds is likely to increase.

The reasons why wounds fail to heal within expected timeframes are complicated and depend on the interplay of multiple influences. Comorbidities, treatment regimens, nutritional status and age may help to impede healing. Chronic wounds are typified by the presence of elevated levels of pro-inflammatory cytokines, proteases and free radicals, continued presence of neutrophils and the absence of activated macrophages (Tarnuzzer and Schultz, 1996).

No specific bacteria have been implicated as the causative agents for retarded healing, but a longitudinal study of chronic venous leg ulcers suggested that a combination of four or more types of organisms was linked to delays (Trengove *et al*, 1996). Recently, biofilms were found to be frequently involved in persistent infections (Costerton *et al*, 1999). Attempts to explain the chronic inflammatory status in wounds had largely focused on host influences but the possible involvement of biofilms has changed the debate.

The role of biofilms in wounds

Microorganisms predominantly exist in nature not in a planktonic state, but as biofilms. They are comprised of single or multiple species adherent to an inert or living surface and enclosed in a self-produced polymeric matrix. Biofilm development is complex and differentiated, and includes initial stages of attachment to the surface and aggregation of cells into complex communities (Hall-Stoodley and Stoodley, 2005). It is now widely accepted that a significant number of human infections involve bacterial biofilms, including endocarditis, cystic fibrosis pneumonia, infections associated with indwelling medical devices and protheses, osteomyelitis, gingivitis and periodontitis (Brady _et al_, 2008; Braxton _et al_, 2005; Hall-Stoodley _et al_, 2004; Hall-Stoodley and Stoodley, 2005; Hall-Stoodley _et al_, 2006; Sbordone and Bortolaia, 2003; Costerton _et al_, 1999).

Biofilms were first linked to wounds when sutures and staples removed from healed surgical wounds were found to be colonised by _S. epidermidis_ (Gristina _et al_, 1985). The colonising bacteria had caused neither infection nor inflammation, demonstrating that biofilms in humans are not necessarily detrimental. The extracellular material surrounding the bacteria was assumed to have assisted persistence by protecting against host defence mechanisms (Gristina _et al_, 1985). The presence of biofilms in wounds was postulated in 2003 (Serralta _et al_, 2001). The demonstration of the ability of a culture of _Pseudomonas aeruginosa_ isolated from a wound to attach and initiate biofilm formation in the laboratory within 10 hours provided some support for this idea (Harrison-Balestra _et al_, 2003). A morphological investigation of material debrided from 12 chronic wounds showed the presence of bacterial biofilms in the necrotic upper layer of seven wounds where it was suggested that repeated seeding of planktonic bacteria from the biofilm biomass perpetuated the host inflammatory response (Ngo _et al_, 2007). A definitive study, using confocal microscopy and scanning electron microscopy, linked biofilms to chronic wounds (30/50) but not acute wounds (1/13); biofilms were located close to the surface of wounds (James _et al_, 2008). A porcine model has provided further evidence of biofilm-associated wound colonisation (Davis _et al_, 2008).

Indirect evidence of the involvement of biofilms in wound chronicity has been deduced from the management of patients with critical limb ischaemia with anti-biofilm strategies. Following sharp debridement and topical use of a patented combination of lactoferrin (which restricts the availability of iron for bacteria) and xylitol (which interferes with the formation of biofilm matrix), the healing rates of 190 patients significantly improved compared with those of a previously published, untreated group (Wolcott and Rhoads, 2008). Recent theories to explain why wounds do not heal have strongly implicated biofilms (Bjarnsholt *et al*, 2008; Wolcott *et al*, 2008).

The involvement of biofilms in infections has considerable clinical implications because these communities are inherently resistant to antimicrobial agents (including antibiotics, disinfectants and germicides) and the host immune response. Silver-based dressings are the most commonly used for infection control. However, while silver exhibits broad-spectrum antibacterial activity, the bactericidal concentration required to eradicate biofilms is 10–100 times higher than that needed to eradicate planktonic cells of *P. aeruginosa* and other pathogens. In addition, it is likely that currently available silver-impregnated dressings do not contain high enough levels of silver to be effective against microbial pathogens growing in biofilms (Bjarnsholt *et al*, 2007), even though one *in vitro* model has demonstrated inhibition by silver-containing dressings (Percival *et al*, 2007). Furthermore, although still relatively rare, silver-resistant bacteria have been reported since 1975 (reviewed in (Percival *et al*, 2005), and toxicity issues have been raised (Cutting *et al*, 2007; Dupuis *et al*, 1985; Trop *et al*, 2006).

Biofilms and honey

There is a large body of *in vitro* evidence for the antibacterial efficacy of honey against planktonic cells that exist in suspension tests and on agar plates, however, there have been relatively few laboratory studies on the sensitivity to honey of biofilms. It has been found that *Leptospermum* and other honeys prevent biofilm formation *in vitro* at concentrations below the MIC (Irish *et al* 2006; Cooper and Jenkins, 2008). Honey may be interferring with the initial mechanisms of biofilm development, such as disrupting processes involved in attachment. Indeed, it has been reported that honey interferes with the ability of *P. aeruginosa* to adhere to surfaces (Lerrer *et al*, 2007), and for *Salmonella enteritidis* to adhere to intestinal epithelial cells *in vitro* (Alnaqdy *et al*, 2005).

Higher concentrations of manuka honey than those needed to prevent biofilm formation were found to be required to cause dispersal of established biofilms of *P. aeruginosa* in laboratory tests (Okhiria *et al*,

2004; Cooper and Jenkins, 2008). These findings have been supported by a study where two honeys (manuka and a Sidr honey from Yemen) were tested against *P. aeruginosa* and *S. aureus* (Alandejani *et al*, 2008). Honey has not yet been shown to eradicate biofilms in patients, but the effect of a honey-impregnated calcium alginate dressing in inhibiting MRSA biofilm in a porcine model was found to be superior to that of either an alginate dressing or a silver hydrofiber dressing (Davis *et al*, 2008).

When honey is used as a wound dressing to clear acute infection the pathogens are, in all probability, growing planktonically. In view of recent publications, it seems likely that the cause of many non-healing wounds may be microbial, even when the classic signs of infection are absent (James *et al*, 2008; Wolcott and Rhoads, 2008). In many instances of patients suffering from chronic wounds, years of conventional treatment had little impact until the commencement of honey dressings which stimulated healing — often after a remarkably short time (reviewed in Molan, 2006). It is reasonable to infer that in at least some instances honey achieved this effect by reducing and/or removing the biofilms that had retarded healing.

One example of biofilm control *in vivo* by active *Leptospermum* honey concerned various measures of dental health, including plaque formation. Plaque is a dental biofilm that has detrimental effects on dental health oral health (Sbordone and Bortolaia, 2003). In a clinical trial the group that chewed a 'honey leather' made from manuka honey had significantly reduced plaque scores compared to the control group (English *et al*, 2004).

Medihoney™ was used prophylactically to prevent infections associated with medical devices (Johnson *et al* 2005) and, although this will be dealt with in *Chapter 7,* it is worth pointing out here that the use of honey instead of mupirocin removes the risk of selecting for mupirocin-resistant strains.

The need to control biofilms in osteomyelitis (Brady *et al*, 2008) and diabetic feet (Davis *et al* 2006) has already been identified. Although further laboratory and clinical investigations are warranted, it is obvious that honey has a role to play in the management of biofilm-associated diseases.

Could 'honey-resistance' become a problem?

It is generally accepted that antibiotic resistance in bacteria is linked to the extensive use of these drugs, particularly for topical antibiotics.

Mupirocin is currently used in nearly 100 different countries, but in Norway, where mupirocin was not licensed, mupirocin-resistant *S. aureus* was not detected (Afset and Mæland, 2003). Comparison of mupirocin susceptibility in MRSA isolated during periods of differing rates of mupirocin usage in an American medical centre demonstrated that stringent administrative control of prescriptions led initially to rapid decline in numbers of mupirocin-resistant MRSA (Walker *et al*, 2004). Similarly, increasing rates of resistance to fusidic acid have been reported (Brown and Thomas, 2002), particularly in dermatology patients (Shah and Mohanraj, 2003; Brown and Wise, 2002). Analysis of prescriptions for fusidic acid and isolations of fusidic acid-resistant *S. aureus* from the community, showed that both had doubled within six years (Mason *et al*, 2003). A retrospective case control study then demonstrated a statistically significant association between fusidic acid resistance in methicillin-sensitive *S. aureus* (MSSA) and exposure to fusidic acid (Mason and Howard, 2004). This was the first confirmation of a causal relationship between the use of a topical antibiotic and increased bacterial resistance. It endorses warnings (Brown and Wise, 2002; Walker *et al*, 2003) that topical antibiotics must be used judiciously. This raises the question — if we see an increased clinical use of honey, will we see the development of honey-resistant pathogens?

This is unlikely to occur for a number of reasons. Firstly, studies investigating the antibacterial activity of *Leptospermum* honey report that the MIC is close to the minimum bactericidal concentration (MBC) (Cooper *et al*, 2002a) (Blair *et al*, manuscript in preparation). This indicates that honey is a bactericidal agent. An antimicrobial compound that has good bactericidal potency, and that maintains tissue concentrations greater than the MIC (or better, the MBC), is effective in minimising the development of antibiotic-resistance (Cazzola *et al*, 2000). Most MIC values reported to date with *Leptospermum* honey (with a level of activity as used in wound care products) have been below 10% v/v. This indicates that dilution factors of more than ten would be needed to reduce concentrations to sub-inhibitory levels, and this is unlikely to occur during clinical use if dressings containing sufficient honey to suit the level of exudate are used (*Chapter 6*). Secondly, compounds with good inhibitory activity against more than one target have lower frequencies of acquired antimicrobial resistance (DeVito *et al*, 2002). Honey is a complex substance made up of over 200 components and it acts against any pathogens present via more than one mechanism. The high sugar content would play a role *in vivo*, as would the low pH and the production of hydrogen peroxide. In the case of active _Leptospermum_ honey, there are additional factors with significant activity, even when this honey is highly diluted. It is also possible that some of the other components in honey interfere with the ability of pathogens to develop resistance to honey. Furthermore, attempts in our laboratories to select for honey-resistant mutants using sub-lethal concentrations of manuka honey have been unsuccessful (data not yet published), although similar experiments to select for antibiotic-resistant strains have been successful. Finally, despite the long history of the extensive medicinal use of honey, no resistance to its antibacterial action has ever been reported. In contrast, resistance to antibiotics was reported almost as soon as they were in common use (Bennett and Parkes, 1944; Bondi and Dietz, 1945; Gallardo, 1945).

Conclusion

The ubiquitous presence of bacteria in wounds can have a myriad of effects. They can be relatively harmless or life threatening, and numerous factors including the health of the host and the characteristics of the microbes can result in a rapid transformation from the innocuous to the extremely menacing. The prevention and treatment of bacterial infections is one of the major concerns of modern wound care. This is a complex field due to the overlapping and interweaved issues associated with nosocomial infections, wound colonisation and biofilms; and these are further complicated by the increasing global emergency of antibiotic-resistance. To address the urgent problem of antibiotic resistance, numerous control programmes have been instigated. It is well accepted that:

- there is a need for a reduction in the use of antibiotics
- more appropriate choices of antibacterial agents and regimens should be instigated
- prevention of cross-infection is paramount
- development of new but effective methods of infection control and required
- development of antibacterial agents with new modes of action is needed.

To at least some degree, an increased clinical use of honey would positively address all of these points.

Honey shows its greatest potential as an agent to significantly reduce the ability of pathogens to establish and maintain infections in wounds. To the best of our knowledge there are no other equally potent, broad-spectrum antimicrobial agents that are as effective against antibiotic-resistant and antibiotic-sensitive pathogens, which inhibit biofilm formation and reduce wound colonisation, while being non-toxic to mammalian cells and having the ability to significantly promote wound healing.

Honey dressings should move from being a 'last resort' to the 'first choice'. There are numerous instances of modern physicians 'resorting' to honey when all conventional treatments have failed, and then seeing rapid and dramatic improvements. Honey dressings should be initiated at the start of patient treatment in various circumstances. Such situations include dressings for burns and ulcers, as well as applying honey prophylactically to surgical wounds and around catheter sites to prevent infection and reduce healing time. A greater initial use of honey would alleviate patient suffering and reduce costs to healthcare systems.

Honey should certainly not be viewed as a panacea. There are cases where it will not achieve complete healing such as where there are malignancies, nutritional deficiencies, congenital abnormalities or circulation problems; there are also issues with keeping it in place and in constant contact with the wound. However, given its potential to positively address many aspects of the overlapping and increasing problems associated with wound infections, honey is grossly under-utilised in modern medicine.

References

Afset JE, Mæland JA (2003) Susceptibility of skin and soft-tissue isolates of *Staphylococcus aureus* and *Streptococcus pyogenes* to topical antibiotics: indications of clonal spread of fusidic acid-resistant *Staphylococcus aureus*. *Scand J Infect Dis* **35**: 84–9

Alandejani T, Marsan JG, Ferris W, Chan F (2008) Effectiveness of honey on *S. aureus* and *P. aeruginosa* biofilms. *Otolaryngol Head Neck Surg* **139**(1): 107

Albrecht MA, Griffith ME, Murray CK, Chung KK, Horvath EE, Ward JA, *et al* (2006) Impact of *Acinetobacter* infection on the mortality of burn patients. *J Am Coll Surg* **203**: 546–50

Alnaqdy A, Al-Jabri A, Al Mahrooqi Z, Nzeako B, Nsanze H (2005) Inhibition effect of honey on the adherence of *Salmonella* to intestinal epithelial cells *in vitro*. *Int J Food Microbiol* **103**: 347–51

Appelgren P, Bjornhagen V, Bragderyd K, Jonsson CE, Ransjo U (2002) A prospective study of infections in burn patients. _Burns_ 28: 39–46

Avdic E, Cosgrove SE (2008) Management and control strategies for community-associated methicillin-resistant _Staphylococcus aureus. Expert Opinion Pharmacother_ 9: 1463–79

Bennett TI, Parkes T (1944) Penicillin in sulphonamide-resistant pneumonias. _Lancet_ 246: 305–8

Bjarnsholt T, Kirketerp-Møller K, Kristiansen S, Phipps R, Nielsen AK, Jensen PØ, et al (2007) Silver against _Pseudomonas aeruginosa_ biofilms. _APMIS_ 115(8): 921–8

Bjarnsholt T, Kirketerp-Møller K, Jensen PØ, Madsen KG, Phipps R, Krogfelt K, et al (2008) Why chronic wounds will not heal: a new hypothesis. _Wound Rep Regen_ 16(1): 2–10

Blaser G, Santos K, Bode U, Vetter H, Simon A (2007) Effect of medical honey on wounds colonised or infected with MRSA. _J Wound Care_ 16(8): 325–8

Bondi A, Dietz CC (1945) Penicillin-resistant Staphylococci. _Proc Soc Exp Biol Med_ 60: 55–8

Bowler PG, Davies BJ, Jones SA (1999) Microbial involvement in chronic wound involvement. _J Wound Care_ 8(5): 216–8

Bowler PG, Duerden BJ, Armstrong DG (2001) Wound microbiology and associated approaches in wound management. _Clin Micro Rev_ 14(2): 244–69

Brady RA, Leid JG, Calhoun JH, Costerton JW, Shirtliff ME (2008) Osteomyelitis and the role of biofilms in chronic infections. _FEMS Immunol Med Microbil_ 52: 13–22

Braxton EE, Ehrlich GD, Hall-Stoodley L, Stoodley P, Veeh R, Fux C, et al (2005) Role of biofilms in neurosurgical device-related infections. _Neurosurg Rev_ 28: 249–55

Brown EM, Thomas P (2002) Fusidic acid resistance in _Staphylococcus aureus_ isolates. _Lancet_ 359: 803

Brown EM, Wise R (2002) Fusidic acid cream for impetigo. _Br Med J_ 324: 1394

Bucknall TE (1980) The effect of local infection upon wound healing: an experimental study. _Br J Surg_ 67: 851–5

Cazzola M, Matera MG, Noschese P (2000) Parenteral antibiotic therapy in the treatment of lower respiratory tract infections. Strategies to minimize the development of antibiotic resistance. _Pulm Pharmacol Therapeutics_ 13: 249–56

Chambers J (2006) Topical manuka honey for MRSA contaminated skin ulcers. _Palliative Med_ 20: 557

Chung HJ, Jeon HS, Sung H, Kim MN, Hong S J (2008) Epidemiological characteristics of methicillin-resistant _Staphylococcus aureus_ isolates from children with eczematous atopic dermatitis lesions. _J Clin Microbiol_ 46: 991–5

Church D, Elsayed S, Reid O, Winston B, Lindsay R (2006) Burn wound infections. _Clini Microbiol Rev_ 19: 403

Cooper RA, Molan PC, Harding KG (1999) Antibacterial activity of honey against strains of *Staphylococcus aureus* from infected wounds. *J Roy Soc Med* **92**: 283–5

Cooper RA, Wigley P, Burton NF (2000) Susceptibility of multiresistant strains of *Burkholderia cepacia* to honey. *Letters Appl Microbiol* **31**: 20–4

Cooper RA, Halas E, Molan PC (2002a) The efficacy of honey in inhibiting strains of *Pseudomonas aeruginosa* from infected burns. *J Burn Care Rehabil* **23**: 366–70

Cooper RA, Molan PC, Harding KG (2002b) The sensitivity to honey of Gram-positive cocci of clinical significance isolated from wounds. *J Appl Microbiol* **93**: 857–63

Cooper RA, Jenkins L (2008) The inhibition of biofilms of *Pseudomonas aeruginosa* with manuka honey. *Wounds* **54**(4): 70

Cosgrove SE, Sakoulas G, Perencevich EN, Schwaber MJ, Karchmer AW, Carmeli Y (2003) Comparison of mortality associated with methicillin-resistant and methicillin-susceptible *Staphylococcus aureus* bacteremia: A meta-analysis. *Clin Infect Dis* **36**: 53–9

Costerton JW, Stewart PS, Greenberg EP (1999) Bacterial biofilms: a common cause of persistent infections. *Science* **284**: 1318–22

Cutting K, White R, Edmonds M (2007) The safety and efficacy of dressings with silver — addressing clinical concerns. *Int Wound J* **4**: 177–84

Davis SC, Martinez BS, Kirsner R (2006) The diabetic foot: the importance of biofilms and wound bed preparation. *Curr Diabetes Reports* **6**(6): 439–45

Davis SC, Ricotti C, Cazzaniga A, Welsh E, Eaglestein WH, Mertz PM (2008) Microscopic and physiologic evidence for biofilm associated wound colonization in vivo. *Wound Rep Regen* **16**(1): 23–9

Davis SC, Rivas Y, Gill J, Perez R, Valdes J, Kirsner R (2008) *The effects of a Leptospermum honey dressing in methicillin-resistant Staphylococcus aureus (MRSA) biofilms using a well established porcine wound infection model*. Poster at Society for Advances in Wound Care symposium held in San Diego, USA

DeVito JA, Mills JA, Liu VG, *et al* (2002) An array of target-specific screening strains for antibacterial discovery. *Nature Biotechnol* **20**: 478–83

Dunford CE, Cooper RA, Molan P, White R (2000) The use of honey in wound management. *Nurs Standard* **15**(1): 63–8

Dunford CE, Hanano R (2004) Acceptability to patients of a honey dressing for non-healing venous leg ulcers. *J Wound Care* **13**(5): 193–7

Dupuis LL, Shear NH, Zuker RM (1985) Hyperpigmentation due to topical application of silver sulfadiazine cream. *J Am Acad Dermatol* **12**: 1112–4

Eddy JJ, Gideonsen MD (2005) Topical honey for diabetic foot ulcers. *J Fam Pract* **54**(6): 533

Edris B, Reed JF, 3rd (2008) MRSA infection in lower extremity wounds. *Int J Low Extrem Wounds* **7**: 28–31

Edwards R, Harding KG (2004) Bacteria and wound healing. *Curr Opin Infect Dis*: **17**(2): 91–6

English HKP, Pack ARC, Molan PC (2004) The effects of manuka honey on plaque and gingivitis: a pilot study. _J Int Acad Periodontol_ 6: 63–7

Eron LJ, Lipsky BA, Low DE, Nathwani D, Tice AD, Vilturo GA (2003) Managing skin and soft tissue infections: expert panel recommendations on key decision points. _J Antimicrob Chemother_ 52(suppl 1): 13–17

Filius PMG, Gyssens IC (2002) Impact of increasing antimicrobial resistance on wound management. _Am J Clin Dermatol_ 3: 1–7

French VM, Cooper RA, Molan PC (2005) The antibacterial activity of honey against coagulase-negative staphylococci. _J Antimicrob Chemother_ 56: 228–31

Gallardo E (1945) Sensitivity of bacteria from infected wounds to penicillin: II. Results in one hundred and twelve cases. _War Med_ 7: 100–3

George NM, Cutting KF (2007) Antibacterial honey (Medihoney™): _in-vitro_ activity against clinical isolates of MRSA, VRE, and other multiresistant gram-negative organisms including _Pseudomonas aeruginosa. Wounds — A Compendium of Clinical Research and Practice_ 19: 231–6

Gethin G, Cowman S (2005) Case series of use of manuka honey in leg ulceration. _Int Wound J_ 2(1): 10–15

Gethin G, Cowman S (2008) Bacteriological changes in sloughy venous leg ulcers treated with manuka honey or hydrogel: an RCT. _J Wound Care_ 17(6): 241–7

Gristina AG, Price JL, Hobgood CD, Webb LX, Costerton JW (1985) Bacterial colonization of percutaneous sutures. _Surgery_ 98(1): 12–19

Hall-Stoodley L, Costerton JW, Stoodley P (2004) Bacterial biofilms: from the natural environment to infectious diseases. _Nature Rev Microbiol_ 2: 95–108

Hall-Stoodley L, Stoodley P (2005) Biofilm formation and dispersal and the transmission of human pathogens. _Trends Microbiol_ 13: 7–10

Hall-Stoodley L, Hu FZ, Gieseke A, et al (2006) Direct detection of bacterial biofilms on the middle-ear mucosa of children with chronic otitis media. _JAMA_ 296: 202–11

Harrison-Balestra C, Cassaniga AL, Davis SC, Mertz PM (2003) A wound-isolated _Pseudomonas aeruginosa_ grows a biofilm _in vitro_ within 10 hours and is visualized by light microscopy. _Dermatol Surg_ 29(6): 631–5

Irish J, Carter D Blair S (2006) _Honey prevents biofilm formation in Staphylococcus aureus._ Proceedings of Eighth Asian Apicultural Association Conference. Perth, Australia

James GA, Swogger E, Wolcott R, Pulcini ED, Secor P, Sestrich J, et al (2008) Biofilms in chronic wounds. _Wound Rep Regen_ 16: 37–44

Johnson DW, van Eps C, Mudge DW, et al (2005) Randomized, controlled trial of topical exit-site application of honey (Medihoney) versus Mupirocin for the prevention of catheter-associated infections in hemodialysis patients. _J Am Soc Nephrol_ 16: 1456–62

Jones SG, Edwards R, Thomas DW (2004) Inflammation and wound healing: the role of bacteria in the immuno-regulation of wound healing. *Int J Low Extrem Wounds* 3(4): 201–8

Kennedy AD, Otto M, Braughton KR, *et al* (2008) Epidemic community-associated methicillin-resistant *Staphylococcus aureus*: Recent clonal expansion and diversification. *Proc Natl Acad Sci USA* 105: 1327–32

Klevens RM, Morrison MA, Nadle J, *et al* (2007) Invasive methicillin-resistant *Staphylococcus aureus* infections in the United States. *JAMA* 298: 1763–71

Kuehnert MJ, Hill HA, Kupronis BA, Tokars JI, Solomon SL, Jernigan DB (2005) Methicillin-resistant *Staphylococcus aureus* hospitalizations, United States. *Emerging Infect Dis* 11: 868–72

Kwakman PHS, Van den Akker JPC, Guclu A, *et al* (2008) Medical-grade honey kills antibiotic-resistant bacteria *in vitro* and eradicates skin colonization. *Clin Infect Dis* 46: 1677–82

Lerrer B, Zinger-Yosovich KD, Avrahami B, Gilboa-Garber N (2007) Honey and royal jelly, like human milk, abrogate lectin-dependent infection-preceding *Pseudomonas aeruginosa* adhesion. *ISME Journal* 1: 149–55

Lusby PE, Coombes AL, Wilkinson JM (2005) Bactericidal activity of different honeys against pathogenic bacteria. *Arch Med Res* 36: 464–7

Lyman IR, Tenery JH, Basson RP (1970) Correlation between decrease in bacterial load and rate of wound healing. *Surg Gynecol Obstet* 130(4): 616–21

McDonnell G, Russell AD (1999) Antiseptics and disinfectants: activity, action, and resistance. *Clin Microbiol Rev* 12: 9–18

Mason BW, Howard AJ, Magee JT (2003) Fusidic acid resistance in community isolates of methicillin-susceptible *Staphylococcus aureus* and fusidic acid prescribing. *J Antimicrob Chemother* 51: 1033–6

Mason BW, Howard AJ (2004) Fusidic acid resistance in community isolates of methicillin susceptible *Staphylococcus aureus* and the use of topical fusidic acid: a retrospective case-control study. *Int J Antimicrob Agents* 23: 300–3

Miller LG, Perdreau-Remington F, Rieg G, Mehdi S, Perlroth J, Bayer AS, *et al* (2005) Necrotizing fasciitis caused by community-associated methicillin-resistant *Staphylococcus aureus* in Los Angeles. *N Engl J Med* 352: 1445–53

Molan PC (2006) The evidence supporting the use of honey as a wound dressing. *Int J Lower Extrem Wounds* 5(1): 40–54

Natarajan S, Williamson D, Grey J, Harding KG, Cooper RA (2001) Healing of an MRSA-colonized, hydroxyurea-induced leg ulcer with honey. *J Dermatol Treatment* 12: 33–6

Ngo Q, Vickery K, Deva AK (2007) Role of biofilms in chronic wounds. *Aus N Z J Surg* 77(suppl. 1): A66

Okhiria O, Henriques A, Burton N, Peters A, Cooper R (2004) *The potential of manuka honey for the disruption of biofilms produced by strains of Pseudomonas aeruginosa isolated from wounds.* Poster presented at the 155th conference of the

Society for General Microbiology, Dublin, Ireland

Paul M, Raz A, Leibovici L, Madar H, Holinger R, Rubinovitch B (2007) Sternal wound infection after coronary artery bypass graft surgery: Validation of existing risk scores. _J Thorac Cardiovasc Surg_ **133**: 397–403

Percival SL, Bowler PG, Dolman J (2007) Antimicrobial activity of silver-containing dressings on wound microorganisms using an _in vitro_ biofilm model. _Int Wound J_ **4**(2): 186–91

Popovich KJ, Hota B (2008) Treatment and prevention of community-associated methicillin-resistant _Staphylococcus aureus_ skin and soft tissue infections. _Dermatol Therapy_ **21**: 167–79

Posnett J, Franks PJ (2008) The burden of chronic wounds in the UK. _Nurs Times_ **104**(3): 44–5

Robson MC, Stenberg BD, Heggars J (1990) Wound healing alterations caused by infection. _Clin Plast Surg_ **17**(3): 485–92

Santucci SG, Gobara S, Santos CR, Fontana C, Levin AS (2003) Infections in a burn intensive care unit: experience of seven years. _J Hosp Infect_ **53**: 6–13

Sbordone L, Bortolaia C (2003) Oral microbial biofilms and plaque-related diseases: microbial communities and their role in the shift from oral health to disease. _Clin Oral Investig_ **7**: 181–8

Serralta VW, Harrison-Belestra C, Cazzaniga AL, Davis SC, Mertz PM (2001) Lifestyles of bacteria in wounds: presence of biofilms? _Wounds_ **13**(1): 29–34

Shah M, Mohanraj M (2003) High levels of fusidic acid-resistant _Staphylococcus aureus_ in dermatology patients. _Br J Dermatol_ **148**: 1018–20

Silla RC, Fong J, Wright J, Wood F (2006) Infection in acute burn wounds following the Bali bombings: A comparative prospective audit. _Burns_ **32**: 139–44

Simon A, Softa K, Wiszniewsky G, Blaser G, Bode U, Fleischhack G (2006) Wound care with antibacterial honey (Medihoney) in pediatric haematology. _Support Care Cancer_ **14**: 91–7

Spellberg B, Powers JH, Brass EP, Miller LG, Edwards JE (2004) Trends in antimicrobial drug development: Implications for the future. _Clin Infect Dis_ **38**: 1279–86

Stone PW, Braccia D, Larson E (2005) Systematic review of economic analyses of health care-associated infections. _Am J Infect Control_ **33**: 501–9

Stryjewski ME, Chambers HF (2008) Skin and soft-tissue infections caused by community-acquired methicillin-resistant _Staphylococcus aureus_. _Clin Infect Dis_ **46**: S368–S377

Tarnuzzer RW, Schultz GS (1996) Biochemical analysis of acute and chronic wound environments. _Wound Rep Regen_ **4**(3): 321–5

Trengove NJ, Stacey MC, McGechie DF, Mata S (1996) Qualitative bacteriology and leg ulcer healing. _J Wound Care_ **5**(6): 277–80

Trop M, Novak M, Rodl S, Hellbom B, Kroell W, Goessler W (2006) Silver-coated dressing Acticoat caused raised liver enzymes and argyria-like symptoms in burn patient. *J Trauma-Injury Infect Crit Care* **60**: 648–52

van der Weyden EA (2003) The use of honey for the treatment of two patients with pressure ulcers. *Br J Comm Nurs* **8**(12) (suppl): S14–S20

Visavadia BG, Honeysett J, Danford MH (2008) Manuka honey dressing: an effective treatment for chronic wounds. *Br J Oral Maxill Surg* **46**: 55–6

Vowden P, Apelqvist J, Moffat C (2008) Wound complexity and healing. In: European Wound Management Association (EWMA) Position Document: *Hard-to-heal wounds: a holistic approach*. MEP Ltd, London: 2–9

Walker ES, Levy F, Shorman M, David G, Abdulla J, Sarubbi FA (2004) A decline in mupirocin resistance in methicillin-resistant *Staphylococcus aureus* accompanied administrative control of prescriptions. *J Clin Microbiol* **42**(6): 2792–5

Walker ES, Vasquez JE, Dula R, Bulllock H, Sarubbi FA (2003) Mupirocin-resistant, methicillin-resistant *Staphylococcus aureus*: does mupirocin remain effective? *Infect Control Hosp Epidemiol* **24**(5): 342–6

Wibbenmeyer L, Danks R, Faucher L, Amelon M, Latenser B, Kealey GP, Herwaldt LA (2006) Prospective analysis of nosocomial infection rates, antibiotic use, and patterns of resistance in a burn population. *J Burn Care Res* **27**: 152–60

Wolcott, RD, Rhoads DD (2008) A study of biofilm-based wound management in subjects with critical ischaemia. *J Wound Care* **17**(4): 145–55

Wolcott RD, Rhoads DD, Dowd SE (2008) Biofilms and chronic wounds. *J Wound Care* **17**(8): 333–41

Yasunaga H, Ide H, Imamura T, Ohe K (2007) Accuracy of economic studies on surgical site infection. *J Hosp Infect* **65**: 102–7

Young MH, Washer L, Malani PN (2008) Surgical site infections in older adults — Epidemiology and management. *Drugs Aging* **25**: 399–414

CHAPTER 5

QUALITY STANDARDS FOR MEDICAL GRADE HONEY

Peter Molan and Chris Hill

Modern clinical practice requires quality assurance of the honey used in wound care, hence the concept of 'medical grade honey' has been adopted.

Honey is primarily produced by a form of agriculture, termed apiculture, rather than gathered from wild hives, but there is little control over its production. Its actual production, drop by drop, is by bees ranging free in the environment over distances of several kilometres to harvest nectar. Bees could bring in potentially harmful materials in nectar from unknown sources. There is further scope for contamination during the collection of the honey combs from the hives and the extraction of the honey. Various measures need to be taken to minimise the risk of such contamination to medical grade honey. Thus, honey suitable for use as an ingredient in a 'medical device' can only be obtained by skilled and experienced apiculturists.

The nature of honey

The Codex Alimentarius produced by the Food and Agriculture Organisation of the United Nations defines honey as, 'the natural sweet substance produced by honey bees from nectar of blossoms, or from secretions of living parts of plants or excretions of plant sucking insects, which honey bees collect, transform and combine with specific substances of their own, store and leave in the honey comb to ripen and mature'. Honey is a highly concentrated solution of a complex mixture of sugars. Depending on the floral source of the nectar, glucose in honey may be at a level where it supersaturates in solution so crystals of glucose monohydrate form and are suspended in the syrupy solution. These will dissolve if honey gets diluted (e.g. by wound exudate), or if it is warmed. The sugars in honey are primarily glucose and fructose, normally with more fructose than glucose, and the sugar composition varies depending on the source of the nectar. The average composition of 490 samples of honey from the USA was found to be 79.6% sugars and 17.2% water (White *et al*, 1962).

Besides glucose crystals, honey may also have other particles suspended in it. There may be particles of wax from the honey comb, pollen from flowers incorporated in the honey or introduced during its extraction, and debris such as bees' knees picked up on the comb in the beehive. The incorporation into wound tissue of particles from honey which are not biodegradable is likely to give a 'foreign body reaction' and lead to a granuloma being formed. The aim of medical grade honey is to remove by filtration as much of the particulate matter as possible. Allergic reactions to honey (reported as food allergies) are rare (Kiistala *et al*, 1995). In about half of the cases, these have been attributed to a reaction to a specific pollen, the rest to bee proteins in honey (Helbling *et al*, 1992; Bauer *et al*, 1996). The content of bee proteins in honey cannot be avoided since the bees add the proteins to the honey as a secretion from the hypopharyngeal gland during collection of nectar and when processing the honey in the hive (Molan, 1996). The content of pollen, however, can be minimised, so the aim in producing medical grade honey should be to have the pollen content as low as possible.

Honey normally contains between 2,000 and 10,000 pollen grains per gram, which is equivalent to 0.006–0.03% w/w of the honey (Malone, 2002); this can be reduced to even lower levels by filtration. Some processors use a heat exchanger to heat the honey for as short a time as possible, thereby decreasing the viscosity of honey and allowing filtration through the finest filters practicable. Heating is also required to dissolve the coarse glucose crystals which form in extracted honey. To avoid coarse crystals of glucose re-forming from uncontrolled crystal growth in the supersaturated solution formed when they have been dissolved by heating, honey for medical use is usually turned into a 'creamed' form by having the crystal growth seeded with a large number of fine crystals of glucose. The subsequent growth of the crystals occurs at 14°C to get well dispersed, small crystals that give honey a smooth texture.

If honey is heated in bulk for processing, excessively long heating may occur. There are adverse effects on honey when it is heated to high temperatures or kept too long at an intermediate temperature:

the enzyme which produces hydrogen peroxide gets inactivated, and toxic substances such as hydroxymethyl furfural (HMF) and 3-deoxyglucosone (3-DG) are formed.

Pollen grains from some species of plants are small and may pass through the finest filters that can be used with such a viscous fluid as honey. (Pollen grains are in the range of 5–200 µm in diameter — medical grade honey is typically filtered though a 50 µm mesh.) The aim with medical grade honey is to minimise both the content of pollen in honey prior to filtration, and the contamination from other particulate matter which may be too small to remove by filtration. This is partly achieved by treating honey as a medical product right at the outset of the process, ensuring that the cleanest handling practices are observed. There are also specific procedures to extract honey from the combs and compliance will minimise the inclusion of pollen and other particulate matter in the extracted honey.

Pollen rarely contaminates the nectar that bees store in honeycomb cells. Some pollen may possibly fall into the nectar held in flowers, but mostly it gets in from the mouth parts of the 'house bees' which process both the nectar and pollen harvested by foraging worker bees. The bulk of the pollen harvested, which is used as a source of protein for the colony, is stored in the brood comb, but some is also stored in pollen cells interspersed with honey cells in the honey comb. When honey is extracted by crushing the combs, or when a 'loosening' device is used before extraction to liquefy manuka honey, which is a thixotropic honey (commonly done by plunging a sheet of needles repeatedly into the comb), the honey becomes contaminated with pollen from any pollen storage cells in the comb. This can be prevented by excluding any honey comb which contains pollen cells when the honey is extracted.

Honey is normally removed from the comb by cutting off the caps from the cells with a knife or some form of mechanical device before centrifuging the comb to get the honey out. The capped surface of the combs has a great deal of pollen on it that has fallen off bees working on the combs, as well as debris from dead bees. Salvaging honey cut off with the 'cappings' by draining or centrifuging the 'cappings' is normal practice but this introduces debris and extra pollen into honey. Such salvaged honey should not be added to the extracted honey being processed for medical grade honey.

The widespread practice in apiculture of re-using the emptied comb for production of the following season's honey crop is another common source of contamination. Pollen remains in the comb, especially in the pollen cells, when the comb is drained or centrifuged. This pollen will end up in the new honey that the bees pack into the comb. Thus, new 'foundation' comb is required in hives each season when medical grade honey is produced.

Safety of honey

Medical devices containing honey are manufactured under the same regulations as any other medical device. Processing of the raw ingredient is also regulated. However, as said above, the actual production of the raw ingredient is done in the wild, so the only quality control is through good beekeeping practices by apiarists. With many thousands of bees out foraging from a hive, nobody knows which plants they are visiting to collect nectar. To identify and avoid potential sources of contamination, beekeepers must be familiar with the sources of nectar available to their bees within a few kilometres of an apiary site. Great care should be taken of the hives in which medical grade honey is produced, and with honey when it is removed and transported for processing.

Risks of contamination by chemicals

Some plants produce toxic nectar and hives should not be placed close enough for bees to visit them at the time of year when nectar or honeydew could be collected. Commonly known sources of toxic honey are rhododendron (*Rhododendron* spp.) and tutu (*Coriaria arborea*), which produce neurotoxins, and vipers bugloss (*Echium vulgare*), which produces an alkaloid which damages the liver. These sorts of toxins would not be expected to affect wound repair and regeneration, but can easily be kept out of honey by good beekeeping practice.

Another potential source of toxic chemicals which could get into honey via nectar collected by bees is residues on plants that have been sprayed with herbicides, insecticides or fungicides. Certified organic honey should have been inspected to ensure that no such contamination could occur. Manuka trees grow as a wild forest so much contamination is unlikely. Beekeepers should inspect apiary sites to ensure that there is no likelihood of bees picking up agricultural chemicals from farmland within flying distance, or where spray drift could occur.

Chemicals used in apiculture are a further cause of contamination. Some beekeepers use benzaldehyde as a bee repellent to get bees off the honey combs as they are removed from the hive. For production of medical grade honey an air blower should be used instead. To control varroa mites, miticide strips are placed in hives at certain times of the year. To avoid any possibility of the miticide getting into honey, the strips should never be used in hives with honey. The same applies to antibiotics used to treat bee diseases, as residues of these in honey used in wound care could encourage the development of antibiotic-resistant strains of bacteria in wounds. In manuka honey there is no risk of antibiotic residues, as New Zealand is free from the bee diseases for which antibiotics are used. A further possible source of contamination is from para-dichlorobenzene (PDCB), which is used to keep wax moths away from emptied honey combs when they are stored in the winter for re-use next season. The risk of this chemical being found in medical grade honey can be avoided by using only new 'foundation' combs each season. Traditionally, foundation is made from wax melted down from emptied honeycomb; because PDCB dissolves in wax, foundations should be made from plastic when producing medical grade honey.

Another possible source of chemical contamination of honey is from the re-use of containers for the extracted honey. When extracted from the comb, medical grade honey should be packed into new drums, with a new food-grade lining, or into new food-grade polyethylene buckets. The drums or buckets should be sealed in such a way that any liquid spilled on them cannot seep into the honey inside or have any means of entering when the seal broken.

One additional chemical problem has become evident with manuka honey. It is common knowledge among apiarists that the unique type of antibacterial activity of manuka honey can be increased by heating or storing it at ambient temperature for years. In the author's opinion, medical grade honey should have a standard for being fresh and unheated, to avoid the possible formation of cytotoxic dicarbonyls when honey is heated. Fresh manuka honey is golden brown in colour, developing a dark brown colour when it has been heated or aged. Thus, it should be easy for users of manuka honey products to see if this standard has been met.

Risks of microbial contamination

The enzymic production of hydrogen peroxide during the ripening of honey in the comb serves to sterilise the honey sealed in the cells of the comb and is capable of killing spores (Molan, 1992). Risks of microbial contamination of honey arise during and after extraction from the comb. Honey commonly contains pollen and yeasts, bacteria, bacterial and fungal spores and fungal hyphae. Unless honey has been recently contaminated with bacteria, the vegetative bacterial cells in it will be dead (Sackett, 1919). The high sugar content of honey is sufficient to achieve this. However, spores introduced into extracted honey are not killed because there is insufficient unbound water available in fully ripened honey for the enzyme that produces hydrogen peroxide to be active (Bang *et al*, 2003). There are risks to patients' health in using honey that has not been sterilised, as honey occasionally contains spores of *Clostridium* (Snowdon and Oliver, 1996). Spores will not germinate in undiluted honey, but this can occur if honey is diluted by wound exudate. They are strict anaerobes and grow only in areas of necrosis, where atmospheric oxygen is excluded. The risks from clostridia growing in wound tissue after being introduced from honey include gangrene and wound botulism.

There is no risk of such infections if the honey used is a wound-care product registered as a 'medical device'. This honey is usually sterilised by gamma-irradiation so that the antibacterial activity of the honey is not destroyed (Molan and Allen, 1996). However, gamma-irradiation does not remove bacteria, it simply kills them. There can still be an inflammatory response to their endotoxins, so a sterile product containing a large number of dead bacteria can be pyrogenic. For this reason, one of the quality standards for medical grade honey should be that the honey contains a low number of bacteria. As the number of bacteria present in honey cannot be counted once the bacteria have been killed (other than an indirect estimate from measurement of pyrogens in honey), the counting has to be done as viable bacteria ('colony-forming units', cfu) in a plate count before it is sterilised. This count is also important for ensuring that a honey sample will be effectively sterilised by the radiation dose utilised, because the dose will have been validated with known bacterial counts. If a higher than expected number of bacteria were to be present, the dose of radiation may not be sufficient to kill all the bacteria.

The cfu counts from honey samples can vary from zero to tens of thousands per gram of honey (Snowdon and Oliver, 1996). Most samples of honey contain detectable levels of yeasts, although yeast counts are commonly below 100 cfu/g (Snowdon and Oliver, 1996). Bacteria do not grow in honey because of the high sugar content, but osmophilic yeasts can grow to high numbers in honey which has a high water content. Medical grade honey should have a specified maximum permitted water content, that is below the level at which osmophilic yeasts can grow. Bacterial spores, particularly those in the *Bacillus* genus, are regularly found in honey (Snowdon and Oliver, 1996). These are the bacteria which are primarily responsible for the colonies that form in a plate count, because species of bacteria which do not form spores will not have survived the high sugar content of honey. The *Bacillus* spores most probably come from dead bees in the hive. Some unpublished work by one of the authors (PM) investigating this possibility supported this hypothesis. Samples of manuka honey sent into a major processor were obtained which had come from beginner and part-time beekeepers. Samples of manuka honey were also obtained from experienced, large-scale beekeeping businesses. Successful beekeeping businesses have to keep their colonies of bees healthy. The plate counts in the samples from the professional beekeepers ranged from 0–50 cfu/g. In the honey from the non-professional beekeepers, the counts were far higher, ranging up to the maximum permitted in honey for sale as a food (100 000 cfu/g). This illustrates the point that honey suitable for medical use cannot be obtained from food stores.

Good apicultural practice in the production of medical grade honey ensures that the honey taken from the hives is protected from contact with soil or wind-blown dust. Combs where the production of honey has not been completed should not be included in honey collected for medical use. This will avoid the growth of yeasts which has a high water content because the bees have not finished drying off the honey.

Other sources of microbial contamination are post-harvest factors that influence any food product. These can be controlled by good manufacturing practices (GMP) where honey is extracted from the combs, filtered and packed in buckets or drums. Sources of contamination include air-borne microbes, process workers, pests such as rodents and insects, equipment and buildings. GMP protocols include: the need for filtered air, with the building under positive pressure so that unfiltered outside air cannot come in; clean outer clothing and hair covering, which does not go outside the clean processing area; scrupulous hand-washing by processing staff; pest management programmes to keep the premises clear of rodents and insects; suitable storage facilities to ensure that honey containers cannot get contaminated. The importance of keeping boxes of honey combs clean when taken from the hives and transported to processing facilities is obvious, as this is clearly a way in which dirt could be introduced into otherwise clean-handling facilities.

The good beekeeping and honey processing practices outlined above minimise the risks arising from using honey in wound-care products, and should be mandatory to the quality standards set for any honey product sold as a 'medical device'. It is mostly up to the manufacturers of 'medical devices' to set the quality standards of the ingredients that they use. The authors are aware that some manufacturers do set such standards, but there are now many honey products coming on the market. Clinicians with concerns about the safety of the honey used should question manufacturers about their standards. *Table 5.1* lists the quality standards set by one company for medical grade honey. As, in the authors' opinion, these standards are achievable, clinicians should expect them to be observed.

Standardising antibacterial activity of honey

At present, the major reason why clinicians choose to use honey for wound care is because of its antibacterial activity. (This may change as they become more aware of other bioactivities of honey, such as its anti-inflammatory activity, its stimulation of autolytic debridement and its stimulation of growth of wound repair tissues.) The potency of the antibacterial activity of honey can vary up to 100-fold (Molan, 1992). For this reason, there is a need to have quality standards with respect to the antibacterial activity of medical grade honey.

There are various ways to assess the potency of antibacterial activity. One is to count the number of bacteria still alive after a set period of exposure of a bacterial culture to a set concentration of the antibacterial agent. Another is to find the minimum concentration of the antibacterial agent that is needed to inhibit the growth of bacterial culture: this is known as the minimum inhibitory concentration (MIC). The most relevant way when treating infected wounds is an agar diffusion assay, as this mimics the antibacterial agent diffusing into infected wound tissues. It also removes the complication of the extent of the antibacterial activity of honeys other than manuka being related in a complex way to the degree of dilution of the sample. This complexity is due to the generation of hydrogen peroxide on dilution, yet there is no hydrogen peroxide detectable in undiluted honey (White and Subser, 1963). The enzyme responsible (glucose

Table 5.1: An example of the quality standards set for medical grade honey

Harvest protocols:

- Risk assessment of each apiary site
- All hives located minimum of 10 km from any intensive horticulture
- All hives have GPS location recorded
- All batches can be traced to site origin
- All hives located minimum 10 km from any intensive horticulture
- All hives have been inspected by a certified apiarist
- All bees removed prior to extraction
- All frames have top/bottom bars scrapped and removed
- All frames have wax cappings removed
- All frames inspected to ensure absence of pollen cells
- All frames inspected to ensure absence of brood cells
- Risk assessment of harvesting and extraction process

Assay:

- Floral purity < 90%
- Foreign matter < 50 microns
- Crystallisation < 200 microns
- Heavy metals < 20 ppm
- Antibacterial activity: MIC < 5% against *Staphylococcus aureus*
- Microbiology < 50 cfu/g
- HMF < 10 mg/kg
- PDCB: zero tolerance
- Antibiotic contamination: zero tolerance
- Broad-spectrum screening for insecticides: zero tolerance
- Non-contamination level confidence 99%

oxidase) does not become active until honey is diluted, the activity of this enzyme increasing as more water becomes available by greater dilution, but at the same time becoming less active as the substrate for its reaction becomes diluted (Bang *et al*, 2003).

The agar diffusion assay gives an easily measured zone of inhibition around the antibacterial agent. The area of this zone is proportional to the potency of the antibacterial activity of the agent. By including in the assay some solutions of a standard antibacterial agent, it is possible to express the antibacterial activity of the agent under test relative to that of a standard. The antibacterial activity of manuka honey used in wound-care products is measured by reference to the standard antiseptic phenol, using an agar diffusion assay (Allen *et al*, 1991). This assay has the enzyme catalase added to the honey to destroy any hydrogen peroxide present, so that the measurement obtained is only of the non-peroxide antibacterial activity which is unique to manuka and jellybush honey. (It is important when carrying out this assay to check that the catalase has sufficient activity by including a non-manuka honey, which has a high activity due to hydrogen peroxide.) If the enzyme has insufficient activity then honeys, other than manuka, will appear to have non-peroxide activity like manuka honey. Different manufacturers set their own quality standards for the antibacterial activity of honey, and users should enquire what these are.

For honey in modern wound management, it is important to make healthcare practitioners aware that, although all honeys share the same basic chemistry, they are not as generic as other antibacterial agents, e.g. silver. Ancient Greek physicians wrote of some types of honey being good for therapeutic use, while others were not (Aristotle, 1910; Gunther, 1934 [reprinted 1959]). However, many modern users of honey are unaware of this ancient wisdom.

There are known to be variances in antibacterial potency and therapeutic benefits between honeys from different floral sources and, in order for there to be meaningful comparative data between clinical trials on honey, it is important for authors to state the specific type of honey used and the level of its antibacterial activity.

Regulatory requirements

Honey and honey dressings sold for use in wound care are classified as a 'medical device'. Directive 2007/47/EC of the European Parliament and of the Council of 5 September 2007, which amended the Council Directive 93/42/EEC of 14 June 1993 concerning medical devices, defines a 'medical device' as:

> any instrument, apparatus, appliance, software, material
> or other article, whether used alone or in combination,

including the software intended by its manufacturer to be used specifically for diagnostic and/or therapeutic purposes and necessary for its proper application, intended by the manufacturer to be used for human beings for the purpose of:

- diagnosis, prevention, monitoring, treatment or alleviation of disease,
- diagnosis, monitoring, treatment, alleviation of or compensation for an injury or handicap,
- investigation, replacement or modification of the anatomy or of a physiological process,
- control of conception,

and which does not achieve its principal intended action in or on the human body by pharmacological, immunological or metabolic means, but which may be assisted in its function by such means.

The Medicines and Healthcare products Regulatory Agency (MHRA) is a body of the UK Government which was set up in 2003 to bring together the functions of the Medicines Control Agency (MCA) and the Medical Devices Agency (MDA).

These include the regulation of medicines and medical devices and equipment used in healthcare and the investigation of harmful incidents. The principal aim of the Agency is to safeguard the public's health. It does this by making sure that medicines and medical devices work properly, perform their intended functions and are acceptably safe.

Is honey safe?

The MHRA advise that no product is 100% safe, because all products that interact with the body have the potential for side-effects. Depending on the nature of the device or medicine, these may be minor, but they may also be serious and therefore warrant extensive clinical evidence to establish the risk factors.

The key questions for the MHRA are:

- do the advantages outweigh the disadvantages of taking the medicine?
- does the medicine do the most good for the least harm for most people who will be taking it?
- are the side-effects acceptable?

A high level of side-effects may be acceptable for a medicine used to treat a life-threatening illness, but not in one used for a common minor ailment. Ultimately, patients and their healthcare professionals have to weigh up the risks and advantages of each medicine or treatment regimen when determining the most appropriate treatment. Decisions are generally based on the product indications, evidence provided from clinical study data, contraindications and patient factors.

It has been concluded that honey is safe to use (Molan, 2005). In over 500 wound care case studies and 140 cases of using honey in ophthalmology, there has been no mention of adverse effects, other than a small increase in pain in some cases. (The pain is caused by the acidity of honey giving a response in nocioceptors which have been sensitised by inflammation.) Honey is generally contraindicated for people with allergies to bee products and venom.

As a wound management product, honey must be tested for:

1. Cytotoxicity
2. Skin sensitisation
3. Skin irritation and where it is used on breached or compromised surfaces
4. Sub-chronic toxicity
5. Genotoxicity.

Honey must also pass the sterilisation validation and stability tests in order to be classed as a 'medical device'.

It is well documented and cited that honey has been used to treat wounds for centuries and, as far as the authors are aware, no harmful side-effects have been documented. However, in a safety-conscious medical devices market there is no room for complacency. For this reason, a medical standard for honey has been established and is constantly being reviewed to achieve improvements. This standard addresses all the risk factors associated with management of bee hives and extraction of honey for wound care.

Healthcare practitioners must be satisfied in all aspects of honey production, safety and efficacy. If these considerations are not fully addressed by the industry, clinicians will not widely accept honey as a credible alternative therapy for wound management. To support this, manufacturers should declare the type of the honey and ensure the relevant standards are being met and honey production is being driven from a 'medical device' perspective.

Risk assessment

The requirements of ISO14971:2007(E) provide manufacturers with a framework to systematically manage risk associated with the use of a 'medical device'. It is the manufacturer's responsibility to fully assess the risk factors of devices it places on the market, and it is generally accepted that risk has two components:

- the probability of the occurrence of harm
- the severity of the consequences of harm.

Honey is accepted as very low risk; it is a natural product consisting of sugars (mainly glucose and fructose), water, enzymes (added by the bees), minerals, vitamins and plant-specific chemicals. It is usually advised to monitor the glucose levels of patients with diabetes when treating them with honey, although as yet no data has emerged to suggest this as a risk factor.

Honey may only be one component of the 'medical device' and it is important to assess the device as a whole and not consider the components separately. The questions that should be asked are: 'What risk factors are associated when honey is combined with other substances?' and, 'Has performance been compromised or improved?'.

Manufacturers must be vigilant over safety and risk assessment and have an ongoing dialogue (documented) with the end users (i.e. patients and clinicians) to identify any potential problems and deal with them quickly and efficiently. The risk management process includes the following four elements:

1. Risk analysis
2. Risk evaluation
3. Risk control
4. Production and post-production information.

With honey, the production starts with the bee-keepers, where high standards are needed to meet the requirements of the 'medical devices' market. Practices have had to be adapted and new considerations introduced in the honey production process. In case of any problems coming to light in the end-product, apiarists are required to have documentation in place which will allow trace-back through extraction and processing to the location of the sites of the hives from which each batch of honey was collected.

Close cooperation between the device manufacturer and honey industry is essential to ensure the continued supply of medical grade honey. Each party needs to understand the requirements and constraints of their particular industry, and the device manufacturer must take all possible steps to ensure the suitability of the honey for use as or in a wound dressing.

Classification

'Medical devices' are characterised by their indications for use. The classification of wound dressings is typically covered by Medical Devices Council Directive 2007/47/EC (previously 93/42/EEC) annex IX Rule 4:

> All non-invasive devices which come into contact with injured skin are:
>
> - in Class I if they are intended to be used as a mechanical barrier, for compression or for absorption of exudate
> - in Class IIb if they are intended to be used for wounds which have breached the dermis and can only heal by secondary intent
> - in Class IIa in all other cases, including devices principally intended to manage the micro-environment of the wound.

Rule 13 states:

> All devices incorporating, as an integral part, a substance which, if used separately, can be considered a medicinal product, as defined in article 1 of Directive 65165/EEC, and which is liable to act on the human body with action ancillary to that of the devices, are in Class III.

It is up to the manufacturer of the device to determine the classification of the device it places on the market and this is based upon the available evidence supporting the indications of the device. There are some substances, e.g. silver, which the MHRA has indicated must be classified as Class III, indicating that they consider silver a medicinal product or one that has an action ancillary to the device. There can be major financial advantages of being able to make a specific claim for a product, as healthcare professionals are far more likely to use a product if it is specifically indicated for the condition they are treating. However, the costs and time factors involved in providing the evidence necessary to get registration as a Class III device are a major barrier to market entry for new products. In addition to the evidence available, manufacturers have to consider the ethical and financial advantages and disadvantages before deciding which classification route is most appropriate.

Typically, the properties of honey in relation to wound management are considered by manufacturers to be:

- antibacterial protection
- hygroscopic, imparting a debridement property
- reduction of malodour
- maintaining a moist wound environment.

In terms of wound management, the claims are not particularly spectacular and do not fully reflect the results experienced by many practitioners, as described throughout this book. However, the claims do adequately reflect the level and quality of clinical data available for honey wound dressings. Given that the type of honey in many published tests is not documented, it is questionable whether generic data is appropriate for some, if not all, honey dressings.

The role of the MHRA

The MHRA has the power to withdraw a product from the market and, in the case of medicines, to suspend production. The agency can also prosecute a manufacturer or distributor if the law has been broken. Regulatory decisions are impartial and based solely on evidence of quality, safety, and efficacy required for each product. There is a wide range of types of 'medical device', and different products are treated differently by the MHRA, which considers the particular characteristics, drawbacks and advantages of each one.

The MHRA works closely with the European regulator, the European Medicines Agency (EMEA), and is recognised as a trusted and independent source of expertise throughout Europe. The MHRA also collaborates with other international regulators, such as the US Food and Drug Administration (FDA), and UK government agencies involved in health care, including the National Patient

Safety Agency (NPSA) and the National Institute for Health and Clinical Excellence (NICE).

Conclusion

Within the past four years, honey (particularly manuka honey) has been accepted as a modern wound management product with increasing evidence supporting its wider usage. While the level of evidence and adoption into mainstream practice still remains relatively low, the efficacy of honey in practice has ensured it has found acceptance in a wide variety of clinical settings. From a medical devices' perspective, it meets the regulatory requirements based on limited claims and safety. New presentations of medical grade honey combined with improved industry standards and targeted quality clinical data will ensure that honey achieves a substantial growth in the global wound management market share.

References

Allen KL, Molan PC, Reid GM (1991) A survey of the antibacterial activity of some New Zealand honeys. *J Pharm Pharmacol* **43**(12): 817–22

Aristotle (1910) *Historia Animalium.* Oxford University, Oxford

Bang LM, Buntting C, Molan PC (2003) The effect of dilution on the rate of hydrogen peroxide production in honey and its implications for wound healing. *J Altern Complement Med* **9**(2): 267–73

Bauer L, Kohlich A, Hirschwehr R, Siemann U, Ebner H, Scheiner O, *et al* (1996) Food allergy to honey: Pollen or bee products? Characterisation of allergenic proteins in honey by means of immunoblotting. *J Allergy Clin Immunol* **97**(1): 65–73

Gunther RT (1934 (Reprinted 1959) *The Greek Herbal of Dioscorides.* Hafner, New York

Helbling A, Peter C, Berchtold E, Bogdanov S, Müller U (1992) Allergy to honey: relation to pollen and honey bee allergy. *Allergy* **47**(1): 41–9

Kiistala R, Hannuksela M, Mäkinen-Kiljunen S, Niinimäki A, Haahtela T (1995) Honey allergy is rare in patients sensitive to pollens. *Allergy* **50**: 844–7

Malone LA (2002) *Literature review on genetically modified plants and bee products.* Ministry of Agriculture and Fisheries, Wellington, New Zealand

Molan PC (1992) The antibacterial activity of honey. 1. The nature of the antibacterial activity. *Bee World* **73**(1): 5–28

Molan PC (1992) The antibacterial activity of honey. 2. Variation in the potency of the antibacterial activity. *Bee World* **73**(2): 59–76

Molan PC (1996) Authenticity of honey. In: Ashurst PR, Dennis MJ, eds. *Food Authentication*. Blackie Academic and Professional, London: 259–303

Molan PC (2005) Mode of action. In: White RJ, Cooper RA, Molan PC, eds. *Honey: A Modern Wound Management Product*. Wounds UK, Aberdeen: 1–23

Molan PC, Allen KL (1996) The effect of gamma-irradiation on the antibacterial activity of honey. *J Pharm Pharmacol* **48**: 1206–9

Sackett WG (1919) Honey as a carrier of intestinal diseases. In: *Bull Colorado State Univ Agric Exp Stn* **252**: 18

Snowdon JA, Oliver DO (1996) Microorganisms in honey. *Int J Food Microbiol* **31**: 1–26

White JW, Riethof ML, Subers MH, Kushnir I (1962) Composition of American honeys. Department of Agriculture Technical Bulletin, US

White JW, Subers MH (1963) Studies on honey Inhibine. 2. A chemical assay. *J Apic Res* **2**(2): 93–100

CHAPTER 6

GUIDELINES FOR THE CLINICAL USE OF HONEY IN WOUND CARE

Julie Betts

The practice of using honey in wound care is not new. While it may be considered an emerging therapy in today's practice, it has been used by mankind for the last 4,500 years as a wound dressing. The recent rediscovery of honey as a dressing for wounds is largely due to the increasing challenge of managing bacteria in wounds, both in relation to managing bacterial burden in chronic wounds whereby host control of bacteria is often less than optimal, and the increasing resistance of bacteria to antibiotics.

Despite the potential benefits of using honey in wound care, healthcare professionals need to be certain that the honey being used is of sufficient standard to provide benefits for patients (*Chapter 5*). Honeys, including manuka, are known to vary in their potency and effect (Cooper, 2005). Therefore, healthcare professionals are obliged to use a honey product that has stringent quality and control mechanisms that identify the activity of honey as part of the manufacturing process. In New Zealand, the antibacterial activity of manuka honey is rated on a unique manuka factor (UMF) scale. For example, UMF 10 is equivalent in antibacterial activity to 10% phenol and is at a level to kill common wound infecting bacteria. All manuka honey branded for use in wound care is tested to ensure the activity of the honey is sufficiently high to kill common wound-infecting bacteria (Yoon and Newlands, 2005). This standardised rating of manuka honey (UMF) provides confidence that honey used in wound care products will be at a level to be effective.

Using honey products in wound care

Several points require consideration when using honey in wound care.

These include branding or classification of honey, sterilisation of the honey product and availability or amount of honey in the product.

Firstly, honey products should be branded according to their activity, for example, UMF rating of above 10 (for manuka honey), or specifically branded for use in wound care. In addition, products should be sterilised by gamma-irradiation, as this does not destroy enzymatic activity of the honey where sterilisation by heating does.

Products should also be registered as a medical device by appropriate authorities (for example, CE or FDA) to ensure that the product meets manufacturing and safety requirements for use as a wound care product. In the case of using liquid honey on wounds, single-use tubes specifically manufactured for use in wound care are recommended in preference to jars of honey. Honey in jars is neither filtered nor sterilised to the degree required to remove contaminants that make it safe to apply to patients' wounds.

Availability of honey to the wound bed is also important. To maximise the benefit of honey, it should ideally be in contact with the wound bed immediately the dressing is applied. If the honey is bound in a dressing, you should be confident that the honey will be released from the dressing as soon as wound exudate is absorbed into the dressing, and also have some guide as to the amount of available honey in the dressing. This is important, as the smaller the amount of honey available in the dressing, the quicker it will be diluted by exudate to the point of being ineffective. A guide to the amount of honey to expect in a dressing is that a 10 x 10 cm dressing should contain approximately 20 ml (25–30 g) of honey (Dunford, 2000; Molan and Betts, 2000, 2004; Gethin, 2007).

Wounds suitable for treatment with honey

Acute and chronic wounds

Honey has been used successfully on a variety of acute and chronic wounds. Molan (2006), in his review of evidence regarding the use of honey as a wound dressing, identified positive outcomes for honey in 17 randomised clinical trials and five controlled trials with a combined total of 2000 participants. Types of wounds with successful outcomes in the review included:

- abscesses

- burns
- donor sites
- graft sites
- infected wounds
- leg ulcers
- pressure ulcers
- surgical wounds
- surgical wound dehiscence.

Authors not included in Molan's review have also reported the use of honey in the following wounds:

- leg ulcers (Gethin and Cowman, 2005; Jull *et al*, 2008; Sare, 2008)
- pressure ulcers (Gunes and Eser, 2007; Hampton, 2007)
- diabetic foot ulcers (Eddy and Gideonsen, 2005)
- infected wounds (Blaser *et al*, 2007).

Additionally, the following wounds have been observed by the author to have positive outcomes from the use of honey:

- boils
- calciphylaxis
- cellulitis
- sinus
- skin tears.

Types of wound tissue

The ability of honey to stimulate cellular processes (debridement, angiogenesis) and to control factors that negatively influence healing (bacteria, inflammation) make it applicable as a dressing for necrotic, sloughy, granulating and epithelialising tissue. The suitability of honey to tissue types that represent the stages of healing suggests that honey has the potential to be a universal dressing. The only consideration would be matching the frequency of dressing change to the level of exudate.

The osmolarity of honey causes interstitial fluid to be drawn into the honey, thus ensuring a constant flow of nutrients and exudate into the wound bed. This works well when honey is in contact with the wound bed, however, in cases where there is a significant distance between the honey and interstitial fluid, as in the case of thick eschar, honey's osmolarity will result in further dehydration of eschar and delay debridement. While this may not be ideal in normal circumstances, it offers a valuable feature in managing ischaemic ulcers, as by dehydrating eschar, honey prevents extension of the ulcer and the development of wet gangrene.

In the author's experience, scoring the eschar with a blade, applying honey in a liquid form and occluding the honey with a film membrane allows the honey to penetrate the eschar to the wound bed below, thereby facilitating debridement.

Malodorous wounds

Malodour in wounds such as fungating tumours can be a challenge to manage. Offensive wound odour is caused by the presence of aerobic and anaerobic bacteria within the wound. Honey controls malodour by both inhibiting bacterial growth and providing an alternative source of fuel (glucose) for bacteria, rather than tissue proteins which cause release of ammonia, amines and sulphur compounds (White and Molan, 2005). The ability of honey to reduce malodour via a two-pronged approach offers advantages for clinicians over existing dressing products. A number of authors have reported cases whereby honey has reduced malodour in difficult to manage wounds (Robson, 2003; van der Weyden, 2003; Ahmed _et al_, 2003; Gethin and Cowman, 2005; Kingsley, 2005). In the author's experience, honey has demonstrated the ability to rapidly deodorise wounds. However, honey needs to be in contact with the wound on a fairly constant basis and this may necessitate twice-daily dressing changes for patients with particularly high levels of wound exudate.

Diabetic wounds

A common question the author has been asked is whether honey can be applied to wounds of patients with diabetes. This seems to be based on the assumption that, as honey contains a large amount of glucose, it has the potential to elevate blood glucose levels when applied to a wound. The ability of honey to elevate blood glucose levels would require that the glucose in the honey be absorbed into the wound bed and the blood stream via the capillary network. While it is appropriate for clinicians to be concerned about the possibility of this phenomenon, it has yet to be demonstrated. Suggested possible reasons for this not being apparent are:

- the rate-limiting absorptive capacity of the capillary bed to absorb sufficient levels of glucose all at once, as determined by the size of the wound
- the constant outflow of exudate from the wound bed, inhibiting the ability of glucose to be in contact with the capillary bed for a sufficient length of time to absorb enough glucose to elevate blood glucose levels
- the standardisation of amount of honey contained in current dressings (approximately 20 mls), and the slow-release nature of the dressings precludes sufficient honey from being exposed to the capillary network in a bolus dose.

In the author's early experience of using honey on wounds of patients with diabetes, close monitoring of blood glucose levels was standard practice to determine whether or not elevated blood glucose levels would occur. Elevated blood glucose levels as a result of using honey dressings was never observed. Consequently, closer monitoring of blood glucose levels when using honey dressings is no longer standard practice. However, in the case of diabetic patients with extensive wounds where a concern may exist regarding possible absorption of glucose, closer monitoring of blood glucose levels is advised. See *Chapter 8* for further information.

How to use honey dressings

Previously, honey for use in wound care was only available in liquid form and was applied to wounds by spreading honey from a jar onto the wound or secondary dressing. The challenge of keeping liquid forms of honey over wounds is not new. The Smith papyrus (2500 BC) documents honey being mixed with grease and lint as a standard wound salve, a method of keeping honey in contact with the wound (Zumla and Lulat, 1989). Recently, the challenge of retaining honey in wounds has been identified by clinicians as a limiting factor in the acceptance of honey as a mainstream dressing in wound care (Lawrence, 1999).

This challenge has not gone unnoticed to manufacturers who have concentrated on developing and providing honey dressings that facilitate close contact of honey with the wound bed for more prolonged periods of time than application of liquid honey allows.

Today, honey dressings generally consist of either honey impregnated into tulle or alginate fibre dressings, or mixed with substances that facilitate the formation of a honey-gel mixture. The choice of which type of honey dressing to apply to a wound depends on the depth of the wound, location and level of exudate.

Honey gel, ointment or single-use tubes

Honey dressings that come in tube formats are either pure honey or a more viscous preparation of honey, where the honey is mixed with wax to increase adhesion of the honey to the wound bed. The pure honey format is recommended for use in sinus or cavity wounds where placement of fibrous dressings might be difficult, or for autolytic debridement of necrotic tissue. The gel or ointment format is recommended for use on burns, surgical wounds and ulcers where adhesion of honey to the wound is more difficult. Generally, honey in tube formats is more suited to low exuding wounds, as when used on highly exuding wounds the honey can get washed into the secondary dressing leaving no honey in contact with the wound bed. The honey should be placed directly in contact with the wound or skin surface (in the case of boils) and covered by a secondary dressing that focuses on exudate management, retention of honey over the wound, and non-adherence to the wound bed. Film membranes, dry non-adherent and foam dressings are suitable options.

Honey-impregnated tulle dressings

Honey-impregnated tulle dressings consist of a synthetic, fine weave non-adherent dressing impregnated with honey. They have little absorptive capacity so are best suited for low exuding and superficial wounds. These dressings are reported to be easy to use, have good retention and removal, and are comfortable (Stephen-Haynes, 2004). Gauze or cotton absorbent dressings are commonly used as a secondary dressing in combination with honey-impregnated tulle dressings.

Honey-impregnated calcium alginate dressings

Honey-impregnated calcium alginate dressings consist of a calcium alginate dressing impregnated with honey, approximately 20 mls in a 10 x 10 cm dressing. They provide the clinical benefits of both alginate dressings and honey. They can be used on low to heavily exuding, superficial and cavity wounds. The honey dressing should be applied directly to the base of the wound to facilitate exposure of honey to the wound bed. In the case of packing a cavity wound, fill the cavity with several layers of the dressing stacking each layer on top of the previous one until the cavity is filled to the level of the surrounding skin. This increases absorbency, fills in the wound deficit and allows continued release of honey into the wound bed for an extended period of time. On superficial wounds, the dressing should extend over the margin of the wound and cover any areas of inflammation. Generally, absorbent gauze dressings or pads are suitable as a secondary dressing, although hydrocolloids and foams have been reported as appropriate secondary dressings (Robson, 2005; Lay-flurrie, 2008).

Again, the level of exudate and how quickly the honey becomes diluted determines the frequency of dressing change. Once the honey has been washed out of the carrier dressing, it should be changed. This may mean dressing changes as frequently as twice a day for heavily exuding wounds, or every three to five days for low exuding wounds. Initially, wounds may need monitoring daily to determine the frequency of dressing change.

Impregnated honey dressings can be used under compression bandaging, as the release of honey occurs over a longer time period.

Honey gel sheet dressing

A recent addition to the market is a honey gel sheet dressing (Medihoney™) (*Figure 6.1*). The gel sheet consists of a mix of honey and sodium alginate, approximately 20 mls in a 10 x 10 cm size dressing. Mixing sodium alginate with honey provides a more solid structure (for the honey) and increased absorbency. The honey is released from the dressing as exudate is drawn into it, in a similar fashion to cadexomer iodine dressings such as Iodosorb® (Smith and Nephew Healthcare). As the dressing absorbs exudate and releases honey, it becomes a gel leaving no dressing residue. The honey gel sheet is pliable and conforms well to uneven wound surfaces. It is suitable for superficial and cavity wounds, including sinus, as it is easily moulded to fill deficits, absorbent and alleviates the risk of leaving dressing residue as the dressing converts to a gel. The gel sheet dressing is recommended for use on light to moderately exuding wounds. Applying several layers of the dressing over the wound will increase absorbency of the dressing. The dressing should be applied directly to the base of the wound, and, in the case of superficial wounds, extend beyond the margins to cover any areas of inflammation. As the dressing becomes diluted by exudate and converts to a gel leaving no non-adherent dressing interface against the wound, the use of gauze or cotton absorbent dressings as secondary dressings is not recommended. Depending on the level of exudate, film-coated low-adherent dressings, film membranes, hydrocolloids and foam dressings are suitable for use with the gel sheet dressing.

Again, the level of exudate and how quickly honey is diluted dictate frequency of dressing change. Once the sheet has been diluted and converted to a gel, the dressing should be changed. These dressings can also be used under compression bandaging as the honey is released over a longer period of time.

The range of honey dressings available enables clinicians to choose a dressing format that is more appropriate for the wound depth and level of exudate. Suitable dressing formats for managing wounds include:

- sinus wounds: a gel, ointment, tube honey or gel sheet dressing

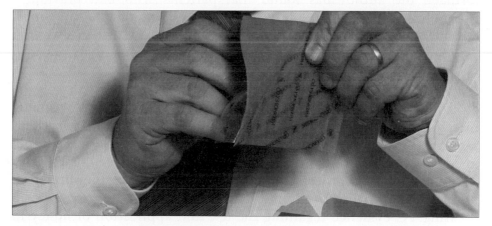

Figure 6.1: The newly-developed honey gel sheet. It is a flexible, non-sticky dressing

- cavity wounds: a honey-impregnated calcium alginate or gel sheet dressing
- superficial wounds: a honey-impregnated tulle dressing or gel sheet dressing.

Suitable honey dressings to match exudate levels are as follows:

- low exudate: gel, ointments and tube honey
- low to moderate exudate: a gel sheet or calcium alginate dressing
- moderate to heavy exudate: a calcium alginate dressing.

Pain can be an issue in applying honey to wounds. The pain caused by honey is due to its acidity. It can vary from a transient stinging in some patients, to marked pain that can last for an hour or more in others. The use of pre-dressing analgesia is useful for patients where pain is anticipated. In situations where honey is causing intense pain which continues for more than an hour, the use of honey should be discontinued. The type of honey dressing applied to the wound can also influence the level of pain experienced. Anecdotal evidence suggests that liquid honey is more painful than other forms. Ointments and gels seem to cause less pain, together with calcium alginate and gel sheet dressings. The author's clinical observation of patients' reported pain with honey dressings indicates a reduction in pain is experienced when honey is released slower from the dressing and over a longer period of time. In evaluating several dressing formats, the author has found that patients who had previously experienced pain with liquid honey and calcium alginate dressings, had marked reduction in pain with the use of a gel sheet dressing. This suggests that pain caused from application of honey to a wound may be influenced by the amount of freely available honey directly in contact with the wound bed.

As with all dressings, precautions should be taken with patients who may have an allergy to components of the dressing. Honey is an easy dressing to use and can be applied to most wounds. It has a role in wound care not only in managing infection, but also in positively influencing cellular processes in healing. The range of honey dressings now available makes honey more acceptable and easier to use as a dressing. As evidence regarding the use and application of honey in wound care continues to grow, so should the acceptance of honey as a mainstream dressing in wound care.

References

Ahmed A, Hoekstra M, Hage J, Karim R (2003) Honey-medicated dressing: transformation of an ancient remedy into modern therapy. _Ann Plast Surg_ **50**(2): 143–8

Blaser G, Santos K, Bode U, Vetter H, Simon A (2007) Effect of medical honey on wounds colonised or infected with MRSA. _J Wound Care_ **16**(8): 325–8

Cooper R (2005) The antimicrobial activity of honey. In: White R, Cooper R, Molan P, eds. _Honey: a modern wound management product_. Wounds UK Publishing, Aberdeen: 24–32

Dunford C (2000) Using honey as a dressing for infected skin lesions. _Nurs Times_ **96**(14): 7–9

Eddy J, Gideonsen M (2005) Topical honey for diabetic foot ulcers. _J Fam Pract_ **54**(6): 533–4

Gethin G (2007) Healing honey. _WIN_ **15**(10): 22–3

Gethin G, Cowman S (2005) Case series of use of manuka honey in leg ulcers. _Int Wound J_ **2**(1): 10–15

Gunes U, Eser I (2007) Effectiveness of a honey dressing for healing pressure ulcers. _JWOCN_(March/April): 184–90

Hampton S (2007) Honey as the new silver dressing. _J Community Nurs_ **21**(11): 45–8

Jull A, Walker N, Parag V, Molan P, Rodgers A, Arroll B, _et al_ (2008) Randomised clinial trial of honey-impregnated dressings for venous leg ulcers. _Br J Surg_ **95**: 178–82

Kingsley A (2005) Practical use of modern honey dressings in chronic wounds. In: White R, Cooper R, Molan P, eds. _Honey: A modern wound management product_. Wounds UK Publishing, Aberdeen: 54–78

Lawrence J (1999) Editorial: Honey and wound bacteria. _J Wound Care_ **8**: 155

Lay-flurrie K (2008) Honey in wound care: effects, clinical application and patient benefit. _Br J Nurs_ (Tissue Viability Supplement) **17**(11): S30–S36

Molan P (2006) The evidence supporting the use of honey as a wound dressing. _Lower Extrem Wounds_ **5**(1): 40–54

Molan P, Betts J (2000) Using honey dressings: the practical considerations. _Nurs Times_ **96**(49): 36–7

Molan P, Betts J (2004) Clinical usage of honey as a wound dressing: an update. _J Wound Care_ **13**(9): 353–7

Robson V (2003) _Leptospermum_ honey used as a debriding agent. _Nurse_ **2**(11): 66–8

Robson V (2005) The use of _Leptospermum_ honey in chronic wound management. In: White R, Cooper R, Molan P, eds. _Honey: A modern wound management product_. Wounds UK Publishing, Aberdeen: 79–88

Sare J (2008) Leg ulcer management with topical medical honey. _Br J Community Nurs_ (Suppl) (September): S22–S31

Stephen-Haynes J (2004) Evaluation of a honey-impregnated tulle dressing in primary care. *Br J Community Nurs* (Suppl) (June): S21–S27

van der Weyden EA (2003) The use of honey for the treatment of two patients with pressure ulcers. *Br J Comm Nurs* 8(12) (Suppl): S14–S20

White R, Molan P (2005) A summary of published clinical research on honey in wound management. In: White R, Cooper R, Molan P, eds. *Honey: A modern wound management product*. Wounds UK Publishing, Aberdeen: 130–42

Yoon Y, Newlands C (2005) Quality standards of medical grade honey. In: White R, Cooper R, Molan P, eds. *Honey: A modern wound management product*. Wounds UK Publishing, Aberdeen: 89–102

Zumla A, Lulat A (1989) Honey — a remedy rediscovered. *J R Soc Med* 82(7): 384–5

CHAPTER 7

USE OF HONEY TO PREVENT INFECTIONS ASSOCIATED WITH MEDICAL DEVICES

Rhianna Miles and David Johnson

The insertion or implantation of medical devices, such as intravascular catheters, has become an indispensable part of contemporary medical practice. The Achilles' heel of such devices is foreign body-related infections, including exit-site infections, bacteraemia and fungaemia. These infections represent the major cause of device removal and are a significant source of morbidity, mortality and excess hospital costs. Strategies for preventing device-related infections have generally focused on cutaneous antisepsis, topical antibiotic application, antibiotic lock solutions and the use of devices coated or impregnated with antimicrobial agents. However, the appearance of antibiotic-resistant microbial isolates has been a significant concern and treatment failures associated with antimicrobial prophylaxis have been reported. Honey is a promising agent in this respect, as it has a low propensity to select for resistant microorganisms and has been shown to exert an antimicrobial action against a broad spectrum of fungi and bacteria, including antibiotic-resistant bacteria, such as methicillin-resistant *Staphylococcus aureus* (MRSA), multi-drug resistant Gram-negative organisms, and vancomycin-resistant enterococci (VRE) (*Chapter 3*). This chapter will review the epidemiology, pathogenesis and prevention of device-related infections, and will focus specifically on the clinical trial evidence pertaining to the use of honey as a chemoprophylaxis agent in medical devices.

Epidemiology of device-related infections

Infections associated with the implantation of medical devices include localised (exit-site, pocket, tunnel) infections and device-related bacteraemias. The most common source of device-related infections is intravascular catheters, which account for 20% of all nosocomial infections (Eggimann, 2007). Reported catheter-related bacteraemia rates range between one and 10 episodes per 1000 catheter-days (Johnson et al, 2002; von Eiff et al, 2005a, b). More than 250,000 central vascular catheter-related bacteraemias and fungaemias occur in the United States each year, with an attributable mortality ranging from 12–25%, and a marginal cost to the healthcare system of $US25,000 per episode (O'Grady et al, 2002; Safdar et al, 2002). Within intensive care units in the USA, there are approximately 80,000 catheter-related bacteraemias each year with the attributable cost per infection estimated at $US34,508–$US56,000, equating to a total annual cost of between $US296 million and $2.3 billion (Mermel, 2000; Rello et al, 2000; Dimick et al, 2001).

Central venous catheterisation is also an increasingly common method of providing rapid, temporary access for the provision of haemodialysis to patients with serious acute or chronic renal failure. Unfortunately, the clinical usefulness of this method is severely limited by the frequent occurrence of bloodstream infections in up to 40% of cases (Marr et al, 1997; Seso et al, 1998; Johnson et al, 2002; Johnson et al, 2005). A number of registry (United States Renal Data System [USRDS], 2003; Polkinghorne et al, 2004) and observational cohort studies (Pisoni, 2002) have indicated that there has been an increasing reliance on haemodialysis catheters in incident haemodialysis patients, ranging from 30% of patients in Europe and Australia to 60% in the United States of America. Recent studies have further suggested that the use of haemodialysis catheters is associated with a 1.5–3-fold increase in both all-cause and infectious mortality (Dhingra et al, 2001; Pastan et al, 2002; Polkinghorne et al, 2004).

Similarly, the use of Tenckhoff catheters for the provision of peritoneal dialysis (PD) to patients with end-stage renal failure has resulted in significant patient morbidity and mortality. PD catheters continue to be complicated by peritonitis despite the introduction of preventative strategies, such as disconnect and double bag systems and topical antibiotic therapy (Strippoli et al, 2004a, b; Wiggins et al, 2007; Wiggins et al, 2008). The incidence of peritonitis varies from one episode per nine to 53 patient months (Wiggins et al, 2007), and the attributable mortality is 5% (Mujais, 2006). Furthermore, approximately 50% of all PD technique failures are due to PD catheter-related infections (Johnson *et al*, 2007a).

Medical device-related infections are caused by a wide variety of microbes, although primarily Gram-positive organisms are the culprit. Among central venous catheters, Gram-positive organisms account for between 61–95% of catheter-related bacteraemias, with *S. aureus* being the predominant cause (Allon, 2004). Gram-negative bacteria are a growing cause of catheter-related bacteraemia, accounting for up to 45% of bacteraemias (including polymicrobial infections). Similarly, Tenckhoff catheter exit-site infections are primarily caused by *S. aureus* (25–85% of cases), which accounts for up to 80% of infection-related catheter loss (Burkart, 1996). Gram-negative organisms (especially *Pseudomonas aeruginosa*, *Escherichia coli*, and *Klebsiella* species) also play a significant role in infection-related catheter loss, accounting for over 10% of peritonitis cases (Bukart, 1996; Mujais, 2006). These bacteria are not prevented by current guidelines for exit-site infection prophylaxis.

Pathogenesis of device-related infections

Medical device contamination most likely occurs as a result of inoculation of skin microorganisms at the time of implantation (von Eiff *et al*, 2005a, b). In the case of intravascular catheters, bacteraemia or fungaemia may occur as a result of the spread of skin organisms along the catheter into the bloodstream, or from contamination and colonisation of the internal and external surfaces of catheters (Dittmer *et al*, 1999; Taal *et al*, 2006; Jaffer *et al*, 2008). Once adhered to the surface, the microorganisms proliferate to form multilayered cell clusters or biofilms, which allow them to evade host defence mechanisms and promote phenotypic resistance to antimicrobial agents (von Eiff *et al*, 2005a, b). Even in the absence of overt infection, microbial colonisation of catheters may engender a chronic inflammatory state which, in turn, increases the risk of erythropoietin-resistant anaemia, malnutrition and cardiovascular disease (McIntyre *et al*, 2004; Johnson *et al*, 2007b). Since the use of tunnelled, cuffed catheters has not been convincingly demonstrated to decrease catheter-related bacteraemia rates (Keohane *et al*, 1983; de Cicco *et al*, 1989; Flowers *et al*, 1989; Timsit *et al*, 1996; Maki *et al*, 1997; Randolph *et al*, 1998; Tokars *et al*, 2002), prophylactic strategies have instead typically focused on topical antimicrobial chemoprophylaxis or antimicrobial catheter lock solutions.

Conventional strategies for preventing device-related infections

Evidence-based clinical practice guidelines for the prevention of catheter-related infections have been published by several groups (O'Grady *et al*, 2002; Piraino *et al*, 2005). The recommended strategies with the strongest supporting evidence include:

- education and training of healthcare providers who insert and maintain catheters
- employing maximal sterile barrier precautions during catheter insertion
- use of needleless catheter connectors
- administration of antibiotics prior to PD catheter insertion
- topical cutaneous antisepsis (von Eiff *et al*, 2005a, b).

Despite these measures, catheter infection rates have remained high leading to heavy reliance upon prophylactic use of antimicrobial agents either applied topically to exit sites, instilled in catheter lock solutions, or impregnated into the devices themselves (Mermel, 2000; O'Grady *et al*, 2002; Taal *et al*, 2006) (*Table 7.1*).

Previous randomised controlled trials have convincingly shown a role for topical mupirocin chemoprophylaxis in preventing catheter-associated infections. Compared with placebo or no treatment, topical mupirocin application was associated with a 7–13-fold reduction in catheter-associated bacteraemias in patients with either non-cuffed, non-tunnelled (Sesso *et al*, 1998) or tunnelled, cuffed haemodialysis catheters (Johnson *et al*, 2002). However, since the publication of these earlier investigations, there has been increasing concern regarding the emergence of mupirocin-resistant staphylococci (Conly and Vas, 2002) and the potential for therapeutic failure (Cookson *et al*, 1990). After introducing mupirocin chemoprophylaxis in our own unit for the prevention of peritoneal dialysis and haemodialysis catheter infections, high-level mupirocin-resistance has emerged, occurring in up to 6% of all staphylococcal isolates. Another group (Lobbedez *et al*, 2004) has not observed an increase in high-level resistance following topical mupirocin administration, but this finding has been contradicted by several reports of disturbing increases in resistance (between 12.4% and 66% of staphylococcal isolates) (Annigeri *et al*, 2001; Conly and Vas, 2002; Perez-Fontan *et al*, 2002; Cavdar *et al*, 2004), particularly with widespread and prolonged mupirocin use

(Conly and Vas, 2002). Furthermore, Perez-Fontan *et al* (2002) have observed a greater incidence of peritoneal dialysis catheter exit-site infections in patients colonised with mupirocin-resistant *S. aureus* compared to those colonised with sensitive organisms, suggesting that the development of mupirocin resistance can have adverse clinical consequences and lead to treatment failures.

Recently, a double-blind, randomised controlled trial of daily exit-site application of gentamicin cream ($n = 67$) versus mupirocin ointment ($n = 66$) found that gentamicin significantly reduced the risk of exit-site infection by 57%, and peritonitis by 35% (Bernardini *et al*, 2005). Based on this study, the International Society of Peritoneal Dialysis (ISPD) guidelines recommend topical antibiotic prophylaxis with either exit-site or nasal mupirocin (applied in either all patients or just nasal *S. aureus* carriers), or daily exit-site gentamicin. However,

Table 7.1: Commonly recommended strategies for reducing the infectious complications of medical devices, such as intravascular catheters (von Eiff et al, 2005a; Eggimann, 2007; O'Grady et al, 2002

Healthcare worker training and education:
- education concerning indications, insertion technique, maintenance and infection control measures
- ensure appropriate nursing staff levels

Regular surveillance for device-related infection

Proper hand hygiene

Administration of intravenous antibiotic prior to peritoneal dialysis catheter insertion

Aseptic technique during device insertion and care

Cutaneous antisepsis (e.g. chlorhexidine, alcohol or an iodophor)

Prompt removal of any device/catheter that is no longer required/essential

Replacement of intravenous administration sets at least every 72 hours

Use of needleless catheter access systems

Antimicrobial prophylactic agents:
- coated or impregnated intravascular devices
- antibiotic lock solutions
- topical antimicrobial agents (e.g. mupirocin, gentamicin cream, etc)
- standardised antibacterial honey

the risks of promoting gentamicin resistance and cumulative toxicity from systemic absorption are likely to be prohibitive in the long term. It would clearly be ideal to develop an alternative safer strategy to either mupirocin or gentamicin for preventing catheter-associated infections without selecting further resistant strains.

Antibiotic locking solutions may also be useful for reducing the frequency of intravascular catheter-associated infections (McIntyre *et al*, 2004; Taal *et al*, 2006; Bleyer, 2007; Jaffer *et al*, 2008). A meta-analysis of seven randomised controlled trials showed that the use of vancomycin lock solution in mostly cancer patients with long-term central venous catheters significantly halved the risk of catheter-related bacteraemias, although the analysis was limited by the presence of trial heterogeneity (Safdar and Maki, 2006). Other antimicrobial agents that may also be effective as catheter lock solutions include 25–40% ethanol (Dannenberg *et al*, 2003; Onland *et al*, 2006), taurolidine (Jurewitsch *et al*, 1998) and minocycline (Bleyer *et al*, 2005). However, concerns about the potential risk of promoting antibiotic resistance have limited the widespread use of this strategy (Mermel, 2007).

Finally, incorporation of antimicrobial agents into medical devices, such as medical polymers (e.g. polymethylmethacrylate) or vascular prostheses, has long been used for the prevention or treatment of bone, soft tissue and vascular graft infections (Moore *et al*, 1981; Marcinko, 1985). More recently, catheters have been impregnated or coated with antimicrobial substances, such as antiseptics (e.g. chlorhexidine) (Haxhe and D'Hoore, 1998; Veenstra *et al*, 1999), metals (e.g. silver) (Boswald *et al*, 1999) or antibiotics (e.g. ampicillin, dicloxacillin, clindamycin, fusidic acid, ciprofloxacin, teicoplanin, cefazolin, minocycline and rifampicin) (von Eiff *et al*, 2005b). A key disadvantage of all of these antimicrobial approaches is the risk of development of microbial resistance against these agents, particularly if the agent used in the catheters is also the first-line drug employed in the therapy of infections associated with that particular medical device (von Eiff *et al*, 2005b). Indeed, the emergence of multi-resistant microorganisms, such as MRSA and VRE, has prompted a more judicious use of antimicrobial agents for chemoprophylaxis and has motivated clinicians and researchers to search for alternative, safer topical antiseptic agents for preventing device-related infections. Such an agent would ideally exhibit broad-spectrum antimicrobial activity without providing selection pressure for resistant microbial strains.

Use of honey as a chemoprophylactic agent for device-related infections

Honey appears to be a promising candidate for preventing device-related infections. The agent has been used from ancient times as a method of accelerating wound healing (Zumla and Lulat, 1989), and is mentioned for healing purposes in the Bible, the Koran and the Torah (Namias, 2003) (*Chapter 1*). Anecdotally, honey has been claimed to reduce inflammation, debride necrotic tissue, reduce oedema, and promote angiogenesis, granulation and epithelialisation (Efem *et al*, 1992). More recently, there have been a number of reports of honey being used successfully as a dressing for wounds, including burns, ulcers, infected surgical wounds, necrotising soft tissue infections, meningococcal wounds and abdominal wound dehiscence (Namias, 2003; Subrahmanyam, 1999; Molan, 2001; Dunford *et al*, 2000). A meta-analysis of seven randomised controlled trials involving the use of honey found that one study had demonstrated that honey was superior to antiseptics and/or systemic antibiotics, and six studies showed it to be superior to conventional and unconventional treatments in maintaining sterility and eradication of infection (Moore *et al*, 2001). However, the generally poor quality of these studies meant that definitve conclusions could not be drawn about the usefulness of honey for superficial wounds or burns.

In laboratory studies, some honeys have been shown to exert an antimicrobial action against a broad spectrum of fungi and bacteria, including antibiotic-resistant bacteria such as MRSA, multi-drug resistant Gram-negative organisms and VRE (Cooper *et al*, 2002a, b) (*Chapter 3*). The reasons for this antibacterial activity include a relatively low water activity (0.56–0.59), low pH (3.2–4.5), the production of hydrogen peroxide on dilution (due to the presence of the enzyme, glucose oxidase) and phytochemical components (including flavonoids and phenolic acids) (Cooper *et al*, 2002b). Despite a considerable accumulated experience of honey use in wound infections, antimicrobial resistance has not yet been reported, thereby making it attractive as a potential means of antimicrobial prophylaxis (Dixon, 2003) (*Chapter 4*).

Since the antimicrobial spectrum of honey is greater than that of most antimicrobial agents used in medical device chemoprophylaxis, and since honey does not appear to result in producing resistant microbial strains, there has been increasing clinical trial interest in this agent for preventing medical device-related infections.

Prevention of haemodialysis catheter infections with honey

The use of honey to prevent haemodialysis catheter infections is a progressing area. Recently, our group published the results of a randomised controlled trial comparing the effect of thrice-weekly exit-site application of honey (Medihoney™) versus mupirocin on infection rates in patients receiving haemodialysis via tunnelled, cuffed central venous catheters (Johnson *et al*, 2005). A total of 101 patients were enrolled between 1 June 2002 and 31 July 2004. No patients were lost to follow-up. Fifty-one patients were randomly allocated to the honey group, while 50 patients received mupirocin. The incidence of catheter-associated bacteraemia in the honey group (0.97 episodes per 1000 catheter-days) was not statistically significantly different from that in the mupirocin group (0.85 episodes per 1000 catheter-days), although these rates were significantly lower than the rate observed in the control group of a previous randomised study in which no topical prophylaxis was applied (10.5 episodes per 1000 catheter-days) (Johnson *et al*, 2002). On univariate and multivariate Cox's proportional hazard model analyses, the type of prophylaxis administered (honey or mupirocin) was not significantly associated with bacteraemia-free survival. No exit-site infections occurred during the study in either group. Honey and mupirocin were both well tolerated. Importantly, 2% of all staphylococcal isolates at the centre had high-level resistance to mupirocin. The median costs of exit-site application for the average life of a haemodialysis catheter were comparable between the honey and mupirocin groups ($13 AUD and $11.10 per patient, respectively). Our group concluded that regular, three times a week, topical exit-site application of standardised antibacterial honey was safe, cost-effective and resulted in a comparable rate of catheter-associated infection to that obtained with topical mupirocin exit-site application in patients with tunnelled, cuffed haemodialysis catheters. The effectiveness of honey against antibiotic-resistant strains of microorganisms and its low likelihood of selecting further resistant strains may mean that honey represents a viable alternative for chemoprophylaxis for haemodialysis catheters. The results of this study are also potentially generalisable to other prosthetic devices, including central venous catheters, Hickman catheters, T-tubes, nephrostomy tubes and peritoneal dialysis (Tenckhoff) catheters.

Following the publication of this study, our unit changed its policy from mupirocin to honey chemoprophylaxis for haemodialysis catheters. Compared with the mupirocin era, median infection-free catheter survival has remained comparable in the honey era (0.58 years [95% CI 0.31–0.85 years] versus 0.59 years [95% CI 0.38–0.81 years], respectively, p = not significant). Several other Australian renal units have also adopted regular topical exit-site application of standardised antibacterial honey as their principal infection prophylaxis strategy in end-stage renal failure patients with haemodialysis catheters.

Prevention of peritoneal dialysis catheter infections with honey

The favourable results for honey chemoprophylaxis in haemodialysis patients has stimulated considerable interest in the potential use of honey chemoprophylaxis in peritoneal dialysis (PD) patients with Tenckhoff catheters. A multicentre, prospective, randomised controlled trial of topical exit-site honey versus nasal eradication of staphylococci for the prevention of Tenckhoff infections in PD patients (Honeypot trial) is currently underway in Australia and New Zealand. The study population includes adults and children with end-stage renal disease who are receiving PD and for whom informed consent is able to be provided. Exclusion criteria include recent (within one month) exit-site infection, peritonitis, or tunnel infection; known hypersensitivity to, or intolerance of, honey or mupirocin; current or recent (within four weeks) treatment with an antibiotic administered by any route; and, nasal carriage of mupirocin-resistant *S. aureus*. Patients will be randomised to one of two treatment groups in equal proportion (*Figure 7.1*). Patients in the experimental intervention arm will receive daily exit-site application of gamma-irradiated, commercially available, pooled antibacterial honeys including *Leptospermum* sp. honey (Medihoney[TM] Antibacterial Wound Gel, Medihoney Pty Ltd, Australia; approximately 10 mg) (*Figure 7.2*). Based upon the recommendations of the CARI

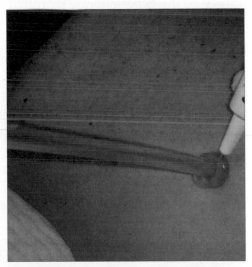

Figure 7.1. Topical exit-site application of standardised antibacterial honey in a peritoneal dialysis patient with a Tenckhoff catheter

Guidelines (74), 2% mupirocin (Glaxo Smith Kline, Australia) will be administered twice-daily to both anterior nares for five consecutive days each month for the duration of the trial for subjects randomised to the control intervention who are identified as staphylococcal carriers. Ascertainment of carriage of *S. aureus* will involve nasal swabs at trial commencement and every six months thereafter. The primary outcome measure will be time to first episode of exit-site infection, tunnel infection or peritonitis (whichever comes first). Secondary outcome measures include:

- time to first episode of peritonitis
- time to first tunnel infection
- time to first exit-site infection
- time to infection-associated catheter removal
- catheter-associated infection rates (including sub-group analyses according to causative organisms)
- occurrence of mupirocin-resistant microbial isolates
- incidence of adverse reactions and costs.

Prospective power calculations indicate that the study will have adequate statistical power (80% probability) to detect a clinically significant increase in infection-free survival from 18 months to 30 months (hazard ratio 0.6) if 185 patients are recruited in each group (370 total), assuming alpha = 0.05, a recruitment period of 24 months, a follow-up period of 12 months, non-compliance rate of 10% and attrition rate of 2% per month (approximately 20% per annum calculated using compounding). It is hoped that the final results will be available in 2011.

Patient population (n = 370)

Inclusion:

- incident or prevalent peritoneal dialysis patients

Exclusion:

- recent (within one month) exit-site infection, peritonitis or tunnel infection
- known hypersensitivity to, or intolerance of, honey or mupirocin
- nasal carriage of mupirocin resistant *S. aureus*

Figure 7.2: Inclusion and exclusion criteria for the Honeypot trial

Conclusions

Medical device-associated infections are a major source of morbidity and mortality. Existing chemoprophylactic strategies are limited by cost and significant concerns regarding the appearance of resistant microbial strains with ensuing treatment failures. There is emerging randomised controlled trial evidence in end-stage renal failure populations that topical, standardised antibacterial honey represents a safe, cheap and effective strategy for preventing catheter-associated infections, without promoting antimicrobial resistance. It is hoped that these preliminary data will foster additional research into the value of honey as a prophylactic agent for preventing infections associated with other medical devices.

References _____

Allon M (2004) Dialysis catheter-related bacteremia: treatment and prophylaxis. *Am J Kidney Dis* 44: 779–91

Annigeri R, Conly J, Vas S, Dedier H, Prakashan KP, Bargman JM, *et al* (2001) Emergence of mupirocin-resistant *Staphylococcus aureus* in chronic peritoneal dialysis patients using mupirocin prophylaxis to prevent exit-site infection. *Perit Dial Int* 21: 554–9

Bernardini J, Bender F, Florio T, *et al* (2005) Randomized, double-blind trial of antibiotic exit site cream for prevention of exit site infection in peritoneal dialysis patients. *J Am Soc Nephrol* 16: 539–45

Bleyer AJ (2007) Use of antimicrobial catheter lock solutions to prevent catheter-related bacteremia. *Clin J Am Soc Nephrol* 2: 1073–8

Bleyer AJ, Mason L, Russell G, Raad II, Sherertz RJ (2005) A randomized, controlled trial of a new vascular catheter flush solution (minocycline-EDTA) in temporary hemodialysis access. *Infect Control Hosp Epidemiol* 26: 520–4

Boswald M, Lugauer S, Regenfus A, *et al* (1999) Reduced rates of catheter-associated infection by use of a new silver-impregnated central venous catheter. *Infection* 27 Suppl 1: S56–S60

Burkart JM (1996) Significance, epidemiology, and prevention of peritoneal dialysis catheter infections. *Perit Dial Int* 16 Suppl 1: S340–6

CARI guidelines (2004) Evidence for peritonitis treatment and prophylaxis: prophylaxis for exit site/tunnel infections using mupirocin. *Nephrology* (Carlton) 9 Suppl 3: S86–S90

Cavdar C, Atay T, Zeybel M, Celik A, Ozder A, Yildiz S, *et al* (2004) Emergence of resistance in staphylococci after long-term mupirocin application in patients on continuous ambulatory peritoneal dialysis. *Adv Perit Dial* **20**: 67–70

Conly JM, Vas S (2002) Increasing mupirocin resistance of *Staphylococcus aureus* in CAPD — should it continue to be used as prophylaxis? *Perit Dial Int* **22**: 649–52

Cookson BD, Lacey RW, Noble WC, Reeves DS, Wise R, Redhead RJ (1990) Mupirocin-resistant *Staphylococcus aureus*. *Lancet* **335**: 1095–6

Cooper RA, Halas E, Molan PC (2002a) The efficacy of honey in inhibiting strains of *Pseudomonas aeruginosa* from infected burns. *J Burn Care Rehabil* **23**: 366–70

Cooper RA, Molan PC, Harding KG (2002b) The sensitivity to honey of Gram-positive cocci of clinical significance isolated from wounds. *J Appl Microbiol* **93**: 857–63

de Cicco M, Panarello G, Chiaradia V, Fracasso A, Veronesi A, Testa V, *et al* (1989) Source and route of microbial colonisation of parenteral nutrition catheters. *Lancet* **2**: 1258–61

Dannenberg C, Bierbach U, Rothe A, Beer J, Korholz D (2003) Ethanol-lock technique in the treatment of bloodstream infections in pediatric oncology patients with broviac catheter. *J Pediatr Hematol Oncol* **25**: 616–21

Dhingra RK, Young EW, Hulbert-Shearon TE, Leavey SF, Port FK (2001) Type of vascular access and mortality in U.S. hemodialysis patients. *Kidney Int* **60(4)**: 1443–51

Dimick JB, Pelz RK, Consunji R, Swoboda SM, Hendrix CW, Lipsett PA (2001) Increased resource use associated with catheter-related bloodstream infection in the surgical intensive care unit. *Arch Surg* **136**: 229–34

Dittmer ID, Sharp D, McNulty CA, Williams AJ, Banks RA (1999) A prospective study of central venous hemodialysis catheter colonization and peripheral bacteremia. *Clin Nephrol* **51**: 34–9

Dixon B (2003) Bacteria can't resist honey. *Lancet Infect Dis* **3**: 116

Dunford C, Cooper R, Molan P (2000) Using honey as a dressing for infected skin lesions. *Nurs Times* **96**: 7–9

Efem SE, Udoh KT, Iwara CI (1992) The antimicrobial spectrum of honey and its clinical significance. *Infection* **20**: 227–9

Eggimann P (2007) Prevention of intravascular catheter infection. *Curr Opin Infect Dis* **20**: 360–9

Flowers RH, Schwenzer KJ, Kopel RF, Fisch MJ, Tucker SI, Farr BM (1989) Efficacy of an attachable subcutaneous cuff for the prevention of intravascular catheter-related infection. A randomized, controlled trial. *JAMA* **261**: 878–83

Haxhe JJ, D'Hoore W (1998) A meta-analysis dealing with the effectiveness of chlorhexidine and silver-sulfadiazine impregnated central venous catheters. *J Hosp Infect* **40**: 166–8

Jaffer Y, Selby NM, Taal MW, Fluck RJ, McIntyre CW (2008) A meta-analysis of hemodialysis catheter locking solutions in the prevention of catheter-related infection. *Am J Kidney Dis* **51**: 233–41

Johnson DW, Chang S, Excell L, Livingston B, Bannister K, McDonald SP (2007a) Peritoneal dialysis. In: McDonald SP, Excell L, eds. ANZDATA Registry Report 2006. Adelaide, South Australia: Australian and New Zealand Dialysis and Transplant Registry: 87–103

Johnson DW, Pollock CA, Macdougall IC (2007b) Erythropoiesis-stimulating agent hyporesponsiveness. _Nephrology_ (Carlton) **12**: 321–30

Johnson DW, MacGinley R, Kay TD, Hawley CM, Campbell SB, Isbel NM, _et al_ (2002) A randomized controlled trial of topical exit site mupirocin application in patients with tunnelled, cuffed haemodialysis catheters. _Nephrol Dial Transplant_ **17**: 1802–7

Johnson DW, van Eps C, Mudge DW, Wiggins KJ, Armstrong K, Hawley CM, _et al_ (2005) Randomized, controlled trial of topical exit-site application of honey (Medihoney) versus mupirocin for the prevention of catheter-associated infections in hemodialysis patients. _J Am Soc Nephrol_ **16**: 1456–62

Jurewitsch B, Lee T, Park J, Jeejeebhoy K (1998) Taurolidine 2% as an antimicrobial lock solution for prevention of recurrent catheter-related bloodstream infections. _J Parenter Enteral Nutr_ **22**: 242–4

Keohane PP, Jones BJ, Attrill H, Cribb A, Northover J, Frost P, _et al_ (1983) Effect of catheter tunnelling and a nutrition nurse on catheter sepsis during parenteral nutrition. A controlled trial. _Lancet_ **2**: 1388–90

Lobbedez T, Gardam M, Dedier H, Burdzy D, Chu M, Izatt S, _et al_ (2004) Routine use of mupirocin at the peritoneal catheter exit site and mupirocin resistance: still low after 7 years. _Nephrol Dial Transplant_ **19**: 3140–3.

Maki DG, Stolz SM, Wheeler S, Mermel LA (1997) Prevention of central venous catheter-related bloodstream infection by use of an antiseptic-impregnated catheter. A randomized, controlled trial. _Ann Intern Med_ **127**: 257–66

Marr KA, Sexton DJ, Conlon PJ, Corey GR, Schwab SJ, Kirkland KB (1997) Catheter-related bacteremia and outcome of attempted catheter salvage in patients undergoing hemodialysis. _Ann Intern Med_ **127**: 275–80

Marcinko DE (1985) Gentamicin-impregnated PMMA beads: an introduction and review. _J Foot Surg_ **24**: 116–21

McIntyre CW, Hulme LJ, Taal M, Fluck RJ (2004) Locking of tunneled hemodialysis catheters with gentamicin and heparin. _Kidney Int_ **66**: 801–5

Mermel LA (2007) Prevention of central venous catheter-related infections: what works other than impregnated or coated catheters? _J Hosp Infect_ **65** Suppl 2: 30–3

Mermel LA (2000) Prevention of intravascular catheter-related infections. _Ann Intern Med_ **132**: 391–402

Molan PC (2001) Potential of honey in the treatment of wounds and burns. _Am J Clin Dermatol_ **2**: 13–9

Moore OA, Smith LA, Campbell F, Seers K, McQuay HJ, Moore RA (2001) Systematic review of the use of honey as a wound dressing. _BMC Complement Altern Med_ **1**: 2

Moore WS, Chvapil M, Seiffert G, Keown K (1981) Development of an infection-resistant vascular prosthesis. *Arch Surg* 116: 1403–7

Mujais S (2006) Microbiology and outcomes of peritonitis in North America. *Kidney Int Suppl* 103: S55-S62

Namias N (2003) Honey in the management of infections. *Surg Infect (Larchmt)* 4: 219–26

Onland W, Shin CE, Fustar S, Rushing T, Wong WY (2006) Ethanol-lock technique for persistent bacteremia of long-term intravascular devices in pediatric patients. *Arch Pediatr Adolesc Med* 160: 1049–53

O'Grady NP, Alexander M, Dellinger EP, Gerberding JL, Heard SO, Maki DG, *et al* (2002) Guidelines for the prevention of intravascular catheter-related infections. Centers for Disease Control and Prevention. *MMWR Recomm Rep* 51: 1–29

Pastan S, Soucie JM, McClellan WM (2002) Vascular access and increased risk of death among hemodialysis patients. *Kidney Int* 62: 620–6

Perez-Fontan M, Rosales M, Rodriguez-Carmona A, Falcon TG, Valdes F (2002) Mupirocin resistance after long-term use for *Staphylococcus aureus* colonization in patients undergoing chronic peritoneal dialysis. *Am J Kidney Dis* 39: 337–41

Piraino B, Bailie GR, Bernardini J, Boeschoten E, Gupta A, Holmes C, *et al* (2005) Peritoneal dialysis-related infections recommendations: 2005 update. *Perit Dial Int* 25: 107–31

Pisoni RL (2002) Vascular access use and outcomes: results from the DOPPS. *Contrib Nephrol* 137: 13–9

Polkinghorne KR, McDonald SP, Atkins RC, Kerr PG (2004) Vascular access and all-cause mortality: a propensity score analysis. *J Am Soc Nephrol* 15: 477–86

Randolph AG, Cook DJ, Gonzales CA, Brun-Buisson C (1998) Tunneling short-term central venous catheters to prevent catheter-related infection: a meta-analysis of randomized, controlled trials. *Crit Care Med* 26: 1452–7

Rello J, Ochagavia A, Sabanes E, Roque M, Mariscal D, Reynaga E, *et al* (2000) Evaluation of outcome of intravenous catheter-related infections in critically ill patients. *Am J Respir Crit Care Med* 162: 1027–30

Sesso R, Barbosa D, Leme IL, Sader H, Canziani ME, Manfredi S, *et al* (1998) *Staphylococcus aureus* prophylaxis in hemodialysis patients using central venous catheter: effect of mupirocin ointment. *J Am Soc Nephrol* 9: 1085–92

Strippoli GF, Tong A, Johnson D, Schena FP, Craig JC (2004a) Catheter type, placement and insertion techniques for preventing peritonitis in peritoneal dialysis patients. *Cochrane Database Syst Rev* CD004680

Strippoli GF, Tong A, Johnson D, Schena FP, Craig JC (2004b) Antimicrobial agents to prevent peritonitis in peritoneal dialysis: a systematic review of randomized controlled trials. *Am J Kidney Dis* 44: 591–603

Safdar N, Kluger DM, Maki DG (2002) A review of risk factors for catheter-related bloodstream infection caused by percutaneously inserted, noncuffed central venous catheters: implications for preventive strategies. _Medicine_ (Baltimore) **81**: 466–79

Safdar N, Maki DG (2006) Use of vancomycin-containing lock or flush solutions for prevention of bloodstream infection associated with central venous access devices: a meta-analysis of prospective, randomized trials. _Clin Infect Dis_ **43**: 474–84

Subrahmanyam M (1999) Early tangential excision and skin grafting of moderate burns is superior to honey dressing: a prospective randomised trial. _Burns_ 1999; **25**: 729–31

Taal MW, Fluck RJ, McIntyre CW (2006) Preventing catheter related infections in haemodialysis patients. _Curr Opin Nephrol Hypertens_ **15**: 599–602

Timsit JF, Sebille V, Farkas JC, Misset B, Martin JB, Chevret S, _et al_ (1996) Effect of subcutaneous tunneling on internal jugular catheter-related sepsis in critically ill patients: a prospective randomized multicenter study. _JAMA_ **276**: 1416–20

Tokars JI, Miller ER, Stein G (2002) New national surveillance system for hemodialysis-associated infections: initial results. _Am J Infect Control_ **30**: 288–95

USRDS (2003) Excerpts from the USRDS 2002 annual data report: Atlas of end-stage renal disease in the United States. _Am J Kidney Dis_ **41**: S1–S260

Veenstra DL, Saint S, Saha S, Lumley T, Sullivan SD (1999) Efficacy of antiseptic-impregnated central venous catheters in preventing catheter-related bloodstream infection: a meta-analysis. _JAMA_ **281**: 261–7

von Eiff C, Jansen B, Kohnen W, Becker K (2005a) Infections associated with medical devices: pathogenesis, management and prophylaxis. _Drugs_ **65**: 179–214

von Eiff C, Kohnen W, Becker K, Jansen B (2005b) Modern strategies in the prevention of implant-associated infections. _Int J Artif Organs_ **28**: 1146–56

Wiggins KJ, Johnson DW, Craig JC, Strippoli GF (2007) Treatment of peritoneal dialysis-associated peritonitis: a systematic review of randomized controlled trials. _Am J Kidney Dis_ **50**: 967–88

Wiggins KJ, Craig JC, Johnson DW, Strippoli GF (2008) Treatment for peritoneal dialysis-associated peritonitis. _Cochrane Database Syst Rev_ CD005284

Zumla A, Lulat A (1989) Honey — a remedy rediscovered. _J R Soc Med_ **82**: 384–5

Chapter 8

The potential use of honey in the treatment of diabetic foot ulcers

Caroline McIntosh and Robert Frykberg

Diabetes mellitus can be defined as a metabolic disorder of multiple aetiology, characterised by chronic hyperglycaemia with disturbances of carbohydrate, fat and protein metabolism (Williams and Pickup, 1999). There are an estimated 2.35 million people living with diabetes in England (Department of Health [DoH] 2007), however, the prevalence of diabetes is predicted to rise to more than 2.5 million in England by 2010 (DoH, 2007). This escalation is thought to be due to an ageing population, sedentary lifestyles and an increasing prevalence of obesity. Indeed, the increasing prevalence of diabetes is a global phenomenon with epidemiological data predicting an increased global prevalence from 171 million in 2000 to 366 million by 2030 (Wild *et al*, 2004).

Foot ulceration is a serious complication of diabetes mellitus, with published data suggesting that between 12–25% of individuals with diabetes will develop a foot ulcer at some stage of their disease (Brem *et al*, 2004). This is concerning given that foot ulcers, among patients with diabetes, are a contributory factor for over 80% of lower limb amputations (Stanaway *et al*, 2007).

An increasing prevalence of diabetes will significantly impact on healthcare services and resources. By 2025, costs of diabetes care are estimated to account for 7–13% of total worldwide healthcare expenditure (International Diabetes Federation [IDF], 2005). The costs associated with diabetic foot disease are not just financial; the personal costs to those affected by the devastating consequences of diabetic foot ulceration (DFU) or lower limb amputation must be considered, as DFU is associated with a reduced quality of life and premature mortality (IDF, 2005). Ribu *et al* 2007 undertook a multi-centre study that compared health-related quality of life in patients with diabetic foot ulcers with a non-ulcerated diabetes group and the general population, and the findings indicated that those with diabetic foot ulcers reported significantly poorer health-related quality of life than those with diabetes without foot ulceration, and the general population.

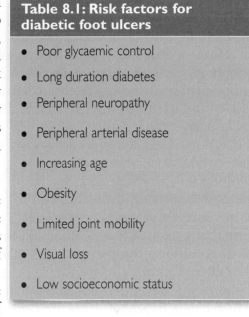

Table 8.1: Risk factors for diabetic foot ulcers

- Poor glycaemic control
- Long duration diabetes
- Peripheral neuropathy
- Peripheral arterial disease
- Increasing age
- Obesity
- Limited joint mobility
- Visual loss
- Low socioeconomic status

Hinchcliffe *et al* (2008) systematically reviewed the literature with regard to the effectiveness of interventions to enhance the healing of chronic diabetic foot ulcers. They concluded that the outcome of management of diabetic foot ulcers was poor, and that there remains uncertainty as to the optimal approaches to ulcer management. The mainstay of treatment involves control of glycaemic levels, vascular control, off-loading/mechanical control, and appropriate local wound care, including wound debridement, management of infection, and exudate management. Honey, as a topical wound care product, has been advocated as a potential therapy in the management of wounds, including diabetic foot ulcers, due to reports of its antimicrobial action, anti-inflammatory action, debriding action, exudate control and stimulation of new tissue (Molan, 2001; McIntosh, 2008). This chapter aims to provide an overview of current concepts in diabetes-related foot ulceration, and the potential role of honey as a topical therapy.

Pathogenesis of diabetic foot ulcers

The cause of diabetes-related foot ulceration is often multifactorial. There are numerous established risk factors that are known to increase the likelihood of foot ulceration (*Table 8.1*).

Perhaps the most significant risk factors for the pathogenesis of diabetic foot disease are peripheral neuropathy (PN) and peripheral arterial disease (PAD).

Peripheral neuropathy

Individuals with diabetes commonly present with autonomic, sensory or motor neuropathy or a combination of the three, collectively known as peripheral polyneuropathy. Peripheral neuropathy is a well established contributory factor to diabetic foot ulceration. Frykberg *et al* (2006) reported that approximately 45–60% of all diabetic ulcerations are purely neuropathic, while up to 45% have neuroischaemic ulceration. The pathophysiology of diabetic neuropathy is not yet fully understood, however, pathophysiological concepts include the depletion of myo-inositol due to the accumulation of sorbitol and fructose, axonal dysfunction, and hyperglycaemia induced generation of advanced glycation end-products (Hilz *et al*, 2000). In the diabetic foot this can manifest as different forms of neuropathy; autonomic, sensory and motor neuropathies (*Table 8.2*).

Zeigler (2008) reported that approximately one in three people with diabetes will develop peripheral polyneuropathy, with distal symmetric sensory or sensorimotor polyneuropathy (DSP) representing the most relevant clinical manifestation. Sensory neuropathy is recognised as the foremost significant causal factor leading to the development of diabetic foot ulceration (Reiber *et al*, 1999; Frykberg *et al*, 2006).

Diabetic neuropathy can give rise to neuropathic pain with between 8–26% of patients with diabetes presenting with painful symptoms, such as persistent or episodic pain (typically worse at night and improved during walking), lancinating stabbing or burning, evoked

Table 8.2: Characteristics associated with diabetic peripheral neuropathy		
Autonomic changes	Sensory changes	Motor changes
Distention of foot veins that are not diminished on elevation	Inability to feel pain	Wasting of intrinsic muscles
Neuropathic oedema recalcitrant to diuretic therapy	Increased risk of unnoticed trauma	Structural deformities
A warm foot due to arteriovenous shunting	Inability to feel temperature sensation	Limited joint mobility
Dry skin prone to fissuring		Elevated foot pressures

pain such as allodynia (pain due to a stimulus that does not normally cause pain), or hyperalgesia (severe pain due to a stimulus that normally causes slight pain) (Zeigler *et al*, 2008). Furthermore, pain associated with diabetic neuropathy exerts a substantial impact on quality of life, particularly by causing sleep interference. Neuropathy is also known to impact on mobility and contribute to the risk of instability and falls, especially in the elderly (Van Schie, 2008).

Foot deformities and structural changes are commonly observed in the diabetic foot, predominantly due to peripheral motor neuropathy, and have been identified as a causal factor in the pathogenesis of diabetic foot ulceration (IDF, 2005). Motor neuropathy can give rise to: intrinsic and extrinsic muscle atrophy; reduced mobility at the ankle (ankle equinus); a high arch profile (cavoid foot type); prominent metatarsal heads; and digital deformities.

Autonomic neuropathy is associated with a long duration of diabetes (Dinh and Veves, 2005), and can give rise to anhydrotic skin that is prone to callus and fissures. This is primarily due to arteriovenous shunting resulting in vasodilation of small vessels and decreased activity of sweat glands (Dinh and Veves, 2005).

The combined effect of the neuropathies outlined above, known as polyneuropathy, can be particularly detrimental to the diabetic foot.

Charcot neuro-osteoarthropathy

Charcot neuro-osteoarthropathy, also known as Charcot foot, has long been recognised as a complication of diabetic PN, which is characterised by joint dislocation, subluxation and pathologic fractures of the foot often giving rise to significant deformities (McInnes and White, 2007). The typical clinical features of Charcot foot are acute unilateral inflammation, increased skin temperature (> 2° C compared to the contralateral foot) and redness, which may have been preceded by a recent minor trauma. McInnes and White (2007) suggested that the pronounced inflammatory reaction associated with Charcot neuro-osteoarthropathy is yet to be fully elucidated. Petrova *et al* (2007) proposed that a systemic inflammatory response may occur. However, in a small sample ($n = 36$), findings suggested that there was a dissociation between the presence of local signs of inflammation, as shown by a normal to slight increase in serum C-reactive protein (CRP, a systemic serologic marker of inflammation). Jeffcoate (2008) highlighted new theories whereby the Charcot foot may be triggered by localised inflammation leading to a vicious cycle of increasing inflammation, increasing expression of pro-inflammatory cytokines and increasing bone breakdown. Regardless of the pathogenesis, individuals with Charcot foot are at great risk of secondary ulceration, particularly over foot deformities that are subjected to abnormal forces during gait.

Peripheral arterial disease

Diabetes mellitus is known to predispose individuals to, and accelerate the progression of peripheral arterial disease (PAD) with reports suggesting the risk of PAD is 20-fold in people with diabetes (Shaw and Bolton, 2001). Peripheral vascular disease in the diabetic patient is characterised by both macrovascular and microvascular changes, including atherosclerosis within leg arteries, and structural and functional changes to the microcirculation which are thought to be primarily due to basement membrane thickening at capillary level and endothelial and smooth muscle dysfunction (Dinh and Veves, 2005). Peripheral arterial disease (ischaemia) is rarely a causative factor for diabetic foot ulceration, but rather an underlying aetiology that will impede wound healing (Frykberg *et al*, 2006). A significant proportion of diabetes-related foot ulcers, 30–50%, dependent on published source, are complicated by the presence of lower limb ischaemia (Frykberg *et al*, 2006; Dinh and Veves, 2005), and the majority of lower extremity amputations in the diabetic population occur due to dysvascularity (Apelqvist *et al*, 1992). It is imperative that all patients with diabetes receive regular vascular assessment to identify dysvascularity at an early stage, so that such adverse outcomes can be avoided. Any limb ischaemia that is compromising wound healing or is considered to be critical, requires referral to the vascular team for revascularisation procedures (Berendt *et al*, 2008).

The typical clinical features of PAD include cold limbs, pallor and/or ischaemic rubor, atrophic, anhydrotic skin and dystrophic toenails (*Figure 8.1*). *Figure 8.1* illustrates lower limb ischaemia with dry 'punched out' ischaemic ulcers to the dorsum and lateral border of the foot.

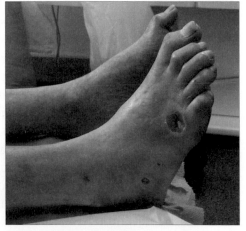

Figure 8.1: Ischaemic ulcerations

Risk factors for delayed ulcer healing

Richard _et al_ (2008) list a number of variables that are known to significantly impact on ulcer healing. These include:

- wound depth
- severity of infection
- neuroischaemic ulcer type
- HbA1c level
- proliferative retinopathy.

Microbial involvement in ulcers is arguably the most important factor that retards healing.

Infection

Immunopathy is common in diabetes due to the associated defects in leukocyte function. Leukocyte phagocytosis has been specifically found to be significantly reduced in patients with poor glycaemic control, which subsequently renders the host more susceptible to infection (Frykberg, 2003). Foot infections are, therefore, commonly observed in individuals with diabetes mellitus. Infection can pose a serious complication in diabetic foot wounds, with infected ulcers taking longer to heal and further increasing the risk of amputation (Stanaway _et al_, 2007) and contributing to morbidity (Richard _et al_, 2008).

Staphylococcus aureus is by far the most frequent pathogen isolated from diabetic foot infections, either as the sole isolate or as a component of mixed infection (Richard _et al_, 2008). Mild infections are often monomicrobial whereas polymicrobial involvement is common in severe diabetic foot infection (Frykberg, 2003).

Infection with methicillin-resistant _S. aureus_ (MRSA) is an escalating problem in both acute and community settings; community-associated MRSA (CA-MRSA) has been described as a clinically significant and virulent pathogen associated with skin and soft-tissue infection, including abscesses and cellulitis (Maeda _et al_, 2008). With regard to diabetic foot ulcer clinics there is some evidence to suggest that MRSA, whether healthcare-associated MRSA (HA-MRSA) or CA-MRSA, is increasingly isolated from diabetic foot ulcers. A study undertaken in diabetic foot ulcer clinics in Manchester, UK, found that the incidence of MRSA from ulcer swabs was 15% (Tentolouris _et al_, 1999), while

Dang *et al* (2003) repeated the study in the same locality in 2003 and found an increase in the incidence of MRSA isolated from wound swabs with figures rising to 30%. Stanaway *et al* (2007) explored the relationship between MRSA isolation from diabetic foot ulcers and nasal MRSA carriage. While the sample size was limited ($n = 65$), findings suggested that nasal MRSA carriage in diabetic patients is a significant risk factor for foot ulcer MRSA infection with 58% of those with positive MRSA ulcer infection having concurrent nasal infection. Furthermore, the authors recognised the need for further research to determine whether eradication of nasal MRSA may reduce MRSA infection in diabetic foot ulcers.

With virulent pathogens and antibiotic resistance becoming a major medical and public health problem, interest in alternative methods to manage infection has arisen. Historically, certain honeys have been known to exert an antibacterial action (*Chapter 1*), with published literature reporting accounts of its inhibitory action against many strains of bacteria, including methicillin-resistant *S. aureus* (MRSA), and rapid clearance of infection from wounds (Molan and Betts, 2004). The antibacterial properties of different honeys vary significantly depending on their floral source (*Chapter 3*).

There is currently limited published evidence that has specifically investigated the effect of honey on infected diabetic foot wounds. Further research is warranted, particularly as published literature has reported an anti-bacterial action of honey against the major wound-infecting species of bacteria. Topical application of honey on diabetic foot ulcers with polymicrobial infection could prove beneficial, but further investigation is required.

In the first reports of the use of honey in treating diabetic foot ulcers, local honeys were used. A cohort of 12 patients with purulent, malodorous wounds were successfully healed with Sudanese honey after antibiotics and antiseptics had been used unsuccessfully (Wadi *et al* 1987). One diabetic patient within the group had a chronic wound extending over the sole of her foot that contained pus and necrotic tissue. After using honey for one week, pus and necrotic tissue were absent and antibiotics were stopped. Honey was continued and a split skin graft applied on week six; amputation was avoided. Honey was used to treat 59 Nigerian patients with wounds and ulcers that had failed to heal with conventional treatments (Efem, 1988). Of the 58 patients successfully treated, four had diabetic ulcers. Again, the use of honey and skin grafting was reported to have been instrumental in avoiding amputation.

A paste prepared by mixing bee propolis, myrrh and honey was used in conjunction with conventional therapies in Saudi Arabia to heal a deep, infected foot ulcer in a patient with diabetes (Lofty et al, 2006). Another reported case where amputation was avoided was in an elderly American patient with two diabetic foot ulcers that had remained unhealed for 14 months, despite optimal care with an orthotic device, antibiotics and surgery. The ulcers were infected with MRSA, vancomycin-resistant enterococci (VRE) and _Pseudomonas_. Topical application of local honey eradicated the pathogens, promoted the formation of healthy granulation tissue within six weeks and healing within six and 12 months, respectively (Eddy and Gideonsen, 2005). A randomised controlled trial to evaluate the effectiveness of honey in treating diabetic foot ulcers is currently in progress in Wisconsin (Eddy, et al, 2008).

Research with modern, licensed products is beginning to be published. In Belgium, an evaluation of a honey-based ointment (L-Mesitran®, Triticum, Netherlands) included 89 patients, of which six were suffering from diabetes. The ulcers were classified using the Wagner scale as five class II and one class III; mean healing time was 29 days, which the authors considered to be short (Vandeputte and van Waeyenberge, 2003). More recently, a neuropathic ulcer on the heel of a patient with diabetes who was suffering from renal impairment was healed within three months with Medihoney™ and no adverse effects on glycaemic control were found (Cadogan, 2008).

Assessment of the diabetic foot

Considerable evidence supports screening all patients with diabetes to identify those at risk of diabetic foot disease (Singh et al, 2005). Regular screening of neurological and vascular status is therefore imperative in the prevention of diabetic foot ulcers.

Neurological screening

International consensus guidelines on the diabetic foot (International Working Group on the Diabetic Foot [IWG], 1999) and the National Institute for Health and Clinical Excellence (NICE, 2004) advocate testing for sensory neuropathy with a 10 g monofilament and 128 Hz tuning fork. The testing of sensory status with a 10 g monofilament is a reliable method to categorise those patients who have an elevated risk of diabetes-related foot problems from those in lower risk categories (Baker *et al*, 2005). The128 Hz tuning fork is another useful modality to identify diabetic PN and predict foot ulceration (Young *et al*, 1994; Garrrow and Boulton, 2006). The neurosthesiometer, as a test for vibration perception threshold, can also discriminate between those at higher risk of foot complications than those at lower risk by quantifying vibration perception. Individuals failing to perceive 25 volts have been shown to have a seven-fold increased risk of foot ulceration (Young *et al*, 1994).

Vascular assessment

NICE (2004) advocate palpation of foot pulses as part of a basic vascular assessment, while the IDF (2005) advise palpation of foot pulses (dorsalis pedis and posterior tibial pulses), plus testing capillary return time and temperature gradient at annual review. However, individuals with diabetes frequently require a more comprehensive vascular assessment to quantify lower limb arterial perfusion, and to identify the presence of arterial risk factors that can lead to the development of arterial disease, for instance, hypertension and dyslipidaemia.

Regular vascular assessment of the lower limbs is important to allow early identification of vascular disease and prompt referral to the vascular team, and subsequent intervention to prevent deterioration.

Established tests to assess vascular status include:

- *Doppler ultrasound:* This is a commonly used screening tool to assess vascular status of the lower limb and foot. Doppler is particularly useful for locating non-palpable pulses and providing audible signals that can inform the practitioner regarding vascular status.
- *Ankle brachial pressure indices (ABPI):* These provide an objective measure of the extent of any PAD in the lower extremities (Marshall, 2004). This test involves measuring systolic blood pressure in all limbs. Pressure in the upper limbs, measured as brachial systolic pressure, should be similar to pressure in the lower limbs, giving a ratio of approximately 1.0 (Vowden and Vowden, 2002).
- Alternative assessment strategies include *toe brachial pressure indices, and transcutaneous oxygen measurement (TcPO2)* which

provides a physiologic measure of tissue oxygenation. TcPO2 measures have been found to be highly predictive of wound healing failure at levels below 25 mmHg (Frykberg et al, 2006).

Referral for vascular consultation should be made in the presence of abnormal, non-invasive findings (_Table 8.3_). Individuals with severe or critical limb ischaemia must be referred to the vascular team urgently in order to save the limb.

Table 8.3: Indications for vascular consultation (Frykberg et al, 2006)	
Non-urgent	Urgent
• Absent foot pulses • ABPI ratio of <0.7 • Toe blood pressures less than 40 mmHg	Critical limb ischaemia defined by: • Ankle pressure <50 mmHg • Toe pressure <30 mmHg • TcPO2 <than 30 mmHg

Clinical features of infection in the diabetic foot

Consensus opinion was gained from a multiprofessional team of wound care experts, utilising a Delphi approach, to identify criteria for infection in diabetic foot wounds (Cutting et al, 2005). _Table 8.4_ lists key markers of infection in the diabetic foot.

Identification of infection in the diabetic foot can prove challenging. Individuals affected by neuropathy may not feel pain associated with an emergent infection, which can result in an episode of infection going unnoticed until it is too late to salvage the foot and partial amputation is required. Furthermore, infection can spread rapidly in the neuroischaemic foot, quickly lead to a limb or life-threatening situation (Frykberg, 2003).

Table 8.4: identifying infection in diabetic foot ulcers (Cutting et al, 2005)
• Cellulitis
• Lymphangitis
• Phlegmon
• Purulent exudate
• Pus/abscess
• Crepitus in the joint
• Erythema
• Increase in exudate volume
• Localised pain
• Malodour
• Probes to bone

Osteomyelitis

Bone infection (osteomyelitis) is a serious complication of pre-existing infected diabetic foot ulcers. It can be recognised clinically by lack of healing despite standard care, including off-loading, and/or visible bone, or ulcers that are found to extend to bone on examination (Hartemann-Heurtier and Senneville (2008). *Figure 8.2* illustrates

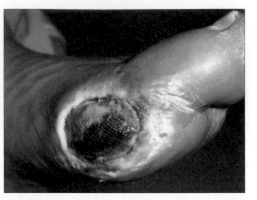

Figure 8.2: Diabetic foot ulcer complicated by osteomyelitis

a diabetic foot ulcer over the first metatarsophalangeal joint complicated by soft tissue infection and osteomyelitis.

Wound assessment

Wound assessment is essential to initially identify the characteristics of the wound and local factors that might impact negatively on the healing process, while ongoing assessment is important to monitor outcomes and establish treatment effectiveness. *Table 8.5* highlights key parameters that should be considered as part of every wound assessment.

Wound classification systems are a useful adjunct to wound assessment, allowing practitioners to grade the wound according to ulcer depth, the presence of infection, osteomyelitis, ischaemia and gangrene.

There are a number of wound classification systems in existence. One classification system specific to diabetic foot ulceration is the University of Texas classification system (Armstrong *et al*, 1998) (*Figure 8.3*).

Management strategies

As suggested by Hinchcliffe *et al* (2008), the outcome of management of diabetic foot ulcers is poor, and there remains uncertainty as to the optimal approaches to ulcer management. Further evidence from robust clinical trials is warranted. However, in the absence of such robust evidence, the management of diabetic foot ulcers involves:

• metabolic control
• vascular control

- off-loading/mechanical control
- elimination of infection
- debridement
- cleansing
- use of appropriate wound dressings to achieve moisture balance and facilitate healing (Hinchliffe *et al*, 2008).

Metabolic control

Glycaemic control is imperative in the prevention of foot ulceration and when trying to facilitate the healing of an established diabetic foot ulcer. The United Kingdom Prospective Diabetes study (UKPDS) (1998) demonstrated that lowering levels of HbA1c (glycosylated haemoglobin) lowers the risk of vascular complications, and suggests that, in practice, patients should aim for near normal levels with HbA1c <7%. The IDF (2005) global guidelines for type 2 diabetes, recommend maintenance of haemoglobin A1C (HbA1c) below 6.5% to minimise the risk of developing complications, for instance, macro and micro-vascular disease, neuropathies and infection, as uncontrolled diabetes is implicated in an increased susceptibility of the host to infection (Frykberg, 2003).

Stage	Grade			
	0	**I**	**II**	**III**
A	Pre- or post-lesion intact	Superficial wound	Penetrating to tendon or capsule	Penetrating to bone or joint
	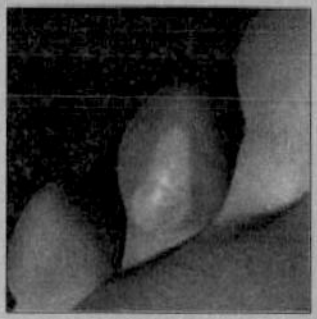	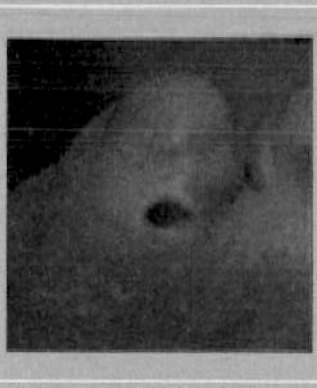	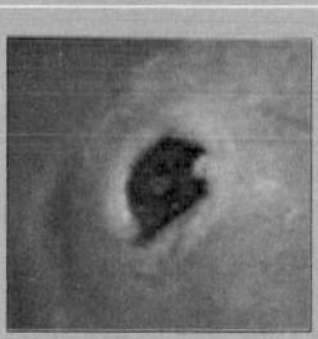	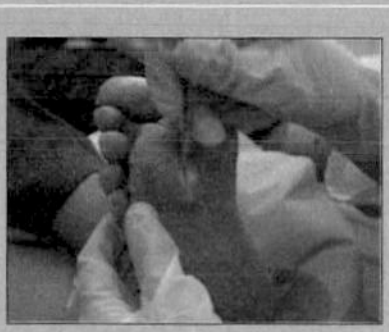
B	+ infection	+ infection	+ infection	+ infection
C	+ ischaemia	+ ischaemia	+ ischaemia	+ ischaemia
D	+ infection and ischaemia	+ infection and ischaemia	+ infection and ischaemia	+ infection and ischaemia

Figure 8.3: University of Texas classifications system (Armstrong *et al*, 1998)

Table 8.5: Factors to consider when assessing a wound (McIntosh and Newton, 2007)

- Wound location

- Wound dimensions (height, width, surface area, depth)

- Nature of the wound bed (necrotic/sloughy/granulating/epithelialising)

- Volume of wound exudate (low/moderate/high)

- Consistency of wound exudate (serous/purulent)

- Wound margins (hyperkeratosis/rolled edges/undermined)

- Pain

- Presence of bony sequestrium or foreign bodies

- Presence of infection

- Condition of the peri-wound skin (e.g. macerated/dermatitis)

- State of surrounding skin (e.g. erythema, inflammation)

Offloading/mechanical control

Offloading and mechanical control of diabetic foot ulcers is essential in both the prevention of primary and secondary ulceration, and to facilitate the healing of active diabetes-related foot ulceration. A systematic review of the literature pertaining to the effectiveness of offloading interventions to heal foot ulcers and reduce plantar pressure in diabetes found evidence to support the use of non-removable devices, with the total contact cast (TCC) touted as the preferred method for off-loading non-infected, neuropathic diabetic foot ulcers on the forefoot (Bus *et al*, 2008). Further studies are required to support the use of other off-loading modalities, such as removable devices, particularly for patients with infected or ischaemic wounds whereby the TCC may be contraindicated.

Management of the Charcot foot depends on the stage of development and complications, such as the presence of ulceration. Treatment is often directed at partial weight-bearing strategies, off-loading high pressure areas or employment of complete immobilisation techniques (McIntosh, 2007).

Wound bed preparation

Brem *et al* (2004) discussed the benefits of sharp debridement of non-viable, infected tissue, including bone, from diabetic foot ulcers (*Table 8.6*), as well as sharp debridement of calluses from the wound periphery, until a border of healthy, bleeding, soft tissue and uninfected bone is created.

Sharp excisional debridement may be undertaken in an outpatient setting by a skilled practitioner, however, more extensive ulcers should be debrided in a theatre setting (Brem *et al*, 2004).

Table 8.6: The benefits of sharp excisional debridement of diabetic foot ulcers (Brem et *al*, 2004)

1. Removes local contaminated bacteria
2. Stimulates healing
3. Documents the absence of hyperkeratotic tissue and tumour
4. Decreases local infection

Wound dressings

There are a plethora of wound dressings available. Dressing selection can prove challenging, particularly given that there is currently no evidence that strongly supports one dressing over another for the management of diabetic foot ulcers.

The following factors should be considered when selecting an appropriate wound dressing (McIntosh and Newton, 2007):

- volume of wound exudate and the ability of the dressing to absorb fluid
- condition of the surrounding skin
- non-adherent properties of the dressing
- patient-related factors such as mobility levels, footwear and desire to bathe
- bacterial burden
- local wound care formularies.

Honey dressings

There is currently limited evidence pertaining to the effect of honey dressings on diabetic foot ulcers, yet there is often a misunderstanding that honey cannot be used on patients with diabetes due to its high sugar concentration. There are no reports in medical literature of hyperglycaemia, electrolyte imbalance or significant irritation to local tissues (Vardi *et al*, 1998). Furthermore, allergic reactions to honey are rare (Molan, 2001).

The potential healing properties of honey have been described in *Chapter 2* and include:

- antibacterial activity
- reduction of inflammation
- deodorising properties
- stimulation of new tissue
- exudate management
- prevention of scarring.

Management of osteomyelitis

Berendt *et al* (2008) stipulated that the principle of treatment for osteomyelitis is to administer antibiotics and maximise their effectiveness at the infected site by removing non-viable soft tissue and accessible necrotic bone during the wound care treatment. *Table 8.7* outlines guidelines for the treatment of diabetic foot osteomyelitis, specifically antibiotic regimens and surgical procedures. The application of topical honey, as an antibacterial, may prove a useful adjunct to antibiotic regimens, particularly for individuals with poor perfusion to the foot, as antibiotics are known to have limited effectiveness in the presence of vascular disease and necrotic tissue, as the amount of antibiotic reaching the wound is reduced (Sheppard, 2005).

Prevention of recurrence

Ulcer recurrence remains a significant problem in diabetes (Bus *et al*, 2008). Care packages for these individuals must be based on preventative strategies.

Prompt access to the specialist multiprofessional team

Any person presenting with an acute diabetic foot problem, including infection, ulceration or Charcot foot, should be urgently referred

Table 8.7: Guidelines for the treatment of diabetic foot osteomyelitis (adapted from Berendt et al, 2008)

Antibiotic regimens	Surgical procedures
Antibiotic regimens should be targeted and narrow spectrum to the infecting bacteria; this can be achieved from the results of bone culture and sensitivity tests	Urgent surgery is required for necrotising fasciitis, deep tissue abscess or gangrene accompanying osteomyelitis
No specific antibiotic has been found to be the most effective for osteomyelitis. Empiric antibiotics should be effective against S. aureus, and MRSA according to local prevalence data	Non-urgent surgery may be indicated if there is significant compromise to soft tissues, the degree of bone involvement is likely to threaten life or limb
There is no data to identify the most effective route of delivery of antibiotics; however, adequate levels of antibiotics in the infected bone can be accomplished with intravenous therapy or highly bio-available oral antibiotics	

to the specialist multiprofessional foot care team to ensure prompt specialised care. A multiprofessional team approach is known to be the most effective means of preventing and treating diabetic foot lesions. Boulton *et al* (2005) undertook a review on the global burden of DFU. Their findings indicated that the establishment of a multiprofessional approach in one centre initiated a 33% reduction in hospital in-patient stay for the complications of DFU. Strategies should therefore be implemented to ensure individuals presenting with diabetic foot disease have rapid access to specialist services when complications arise.

Skin and nail care

Individuals with diabetes are more susceptible to fungal infection of the skin and nails. Onychomycosis (fungal infection of the toenails) affects approximately 34% of patients with diabetes (Gupta *et al*, 1998), and can lead to thickened, brittle nails. If left untreated, this can lead to localised fungal infection of the skin, or subungual ulceration (ulceration under the nail plate) if the nail becomes excessively thickened. Evidence from randomised controlled trials has demonstrated the benefit of regular podiatry care for skin and nail pathologies in the prevention of diabetic foot ulcers and amputation (Plank *et al*, 2003; Ronnemaa *et al*, 1997). All patients with diabetes should receive regular podiatry intervention, particularly when skin or nail pathologies are present to minimise the risk of adverse outcomes. Sensitivity of *Candida* (Irish *et al*, 2006) and dermatophytes (Brady *et al*, 1996) to honey suggest a possible role in controlling fungal foot infections.

Footwear

Therapeutic footwear can be beneficial in the prevention of primary or secondary plantar ulceration in the at-risk patient with diabetes. To achieve effective reduction of peak plantar pressures, custom-moulded insoles should be incorporated in the therapeutic footwear following appropriate assessment, assuming the shoes can accommodate such a device. Extra-depth footwear may not always be sufficient to accommodate significant foot deformity and, in such cases, custom-made footwear is required (Bus *et al*, 2008).

Education/psychosocial issues

The psychological aspect of living with a chronic disease, such as diabetes mellitus, plays an important role in the overall management of the disease process (Price 2008) and should, therefore, be considered as part of any holistic patient-centred care plan. Education on its own will not lead to behaviour change; indeed, Price (2008) suggested that key factors to consider when structuring behaviour change programmes include a readiness to change, confidence in having the necessary skills and family support.

Conclusion

The prevention and management of diabetes-related foot ulceration remains a challenging area of clinical practice. Despite a wealth of published literature in this area, there remains a dearth of scientific evidence to establish the most effective interventions to enhance the healing of chronic diabetic foot ulcers. As suggested by Hinchcliffe *et al* (2008), the outcome of management of diabetic foot ulcers is poor and further research is warranted to address this gap in the evidence base. Honey dressings may have a positive role in the management of diabetic foot ulcers, particularly in the management of soft tissue infection, including MRSA, debridement of slough, odour control and exudate management. One of the author's (RF) own anecdotal experience with an active *Leptospermum* calcium alginate dressing (Medihoney™, Derma Sciences Inc., New Jersey) has indeed shown that honey can expedite healing of such lesions through control of superficial colonisation and promotion of autolytic debridement of slough. Furthermore, the ability of these dressings to effectively manage exudation has allowed for less frequent dressing changes. When appropriate, honey dressings can be applied under a total contact cast and changed at weekly intervals. Nonetheless, controlled clinical trials are required to establish the true potential of honey as a topical therapy in the management of diabetic foot ulceration.

References

Apelqvist J, Larsson J, Agardh CD (1992) Medical risk factors in diabetic patients with foot ulcers and severe peripheral vascular disease and their influence on outcome. *J Diabetes Complications* 6(3): 167–74

Armstrong DG, Lavery LA, Harkless LB (1998) Validation of a diabetic wound classification system. *Diabetes Care* 21(5): 855–9

Baker N, Murali-Krishnan S, Rayman G (2005) A user's guide to foot screening. Part 1: Peripheral neuropathy. *Diabetic Foot* 8(1): 28–37

Bale S, Tebble N, Price P (2004) A topical metronidazole gel used to treat malodorous wounds. *Br J Nurs* (Tissue Viability Supplement) 13(11): S4–S11

Berendt AR, Peters EJG, Bakker K, *et al* (2008) Specific guidelines for treatment of diabetic foot osteomyelitis. *Diabetes Metab Res Rev* 24(Suppl 1): S190–S191

Boulton AJM, Vileikyte L, Ragnarson-Tennvall G, Apelqvist J (2005) The global burden of diabetic foot disease. *Lancet* 366: 1719–23

Brady NF, Molan PC, Harfoot CG (1996) The sensitivity of dermatophytes to the antimicrobial activity of manuka honey and other honey. *Pharm Sci* 2: 1–3

Brem H, Sheehan P, Boulton AJM (2004) Protocol for treatment of diabetic foot ulcers. *Am J Surg* 187(Suppl): 1s–10s

Bus SA, Valk GD, Van Deursen RW (2008) Specific guidelines on footwear and offloading. *Diabetes Metab Res Rev* 24(Suppl 1): S192–S193

Cadogan J (2008) The use of honey to treat an ulcer on the heel of a person with diabetes. *Diabetic Foot* 11(1): 43–5

Cutting KF, White RJ, Mahoney P, *et al* (2005) Understanding wound infection. In: European Wound Management Association (EWMA) Position Document:

Identifying Criteria for Wound Infection. MEP Ltd, London: 2–5

Dang CN, Prasad YDM, Boulton AJM, *et al* (2003) Methicillin-resistant *Staphylococcus aureus* in the diabetic foot clinic: a worsening problem. *Diabetes Med* 20: 159–61

Department of Health (2001) National service framework for diabetes: standards. DoH, London. Available online at: www.dh.gov.uk/ PublicationsAndStatistics/Publications/PublicationsPolicyAndGuidance/ PublicationsPolicyAndGuidanceArticle/fs/en?CONTENT_ ID=4002951andchk=09Kkz1 [accessed 01/09/08]

Department of Health (2007) *About Diabetes.* DoH, London. Available online at: www.dh.gov.uk/en/Policyandguidance/Healthandsocialcaretopics/Diabetes/ DH_074762 [accessed 02/09/08]

Dinh TL, Veves A (2005) A review of the mechanisms implicated in the pathogenesis of the diabetic foot. *Lower Extrem Wounds* 4(3): 154–9

Eddy JJ, Gideonsen MD (2005)Topical honey for diabetic foot ulcers. *J Fam Pract* 54(6): 533–5

Eddy JJ, Gideonsen MD, Mack GP (2008) Practical considerations of using topical honey for neuropathic foot ulcers: a review. *Wisconsin Med J* 107: 187–90

Efem AEE (1988) Clinical observations on the wound healing properties of honey. *Br J Surg* 75: 679–81

Frykberg RG (2003) An evidence-based approach to diabetic foot infections. *Am J Surg* 186/5A: 44s–54s

Frykberg RG, Zgonis T, Armstrong DG, *et al* (2006) Diabetic foot disorders: a clinical practice guideline. *J Foot Ankle Surg* 45(5)(Supp): 1–65

Garrrow AP, Boulton AJ (2006) Vibration Perception Testing — a valuable assessment of neural dysfunction in people with diabetes. *Diabetic Metab Res Rev* 22(5): 411–9

Gupta AK, Konnikov N, MacDonald P, *et al* (1998) Prevalence and epidemiology of toenail onychomycosis in diabetic subjects: a multicentre survey. *Br J Dermatol* 139: 665–71

Hilz MJ, Marthol H, Neundörfer B (2000) Diabetic somatic polyneuropathy. Pathogenesis, clinical manifestations and therapeutic concepts. *Fortschr Neurol Psychiatr* 68(6): 278-88

Hartemann-Heurtier A, Senneville E (2008) Diabetic foot osteomyelitis. *Diabetes Metab* 34: 87–95

Hinchcliffe RJ, Valk GD, Apelqvist J, *et al* (2008) A systematic review of the effectiveness of interventions to enhance the healing of chronic ulcers of the foot in diabetes. *Diabetes Metab Res Rev* 24(Suppl 1): S119–S144

International Diabetes Federation (2005) Clinical Guidelines Task Force (2005) Global Guidance for Type 2 diabetes. IDF, Brussels

International Working Group on the Diabetic Foot (1999) *International Consensus on the Diabetic Foot.* IWG, Amsterdam

Irish J, Carter DA, Shokohi T, Blair SE (2006) Honey has an antifungal effect against _Candida_ species. _Med Mycol_ **44**(3): 289–91

Jeffcoate WJ (2008) Charcot neuro-osteoarthropathy. _Diabetes Metab Res Rev_ **24**(Suppl 1): S62–S65

Lee G, Anand SC, Rajendran S, _et al_ (2006) Overview of current practice and future trends in the evaluation of dressings for malodorous wounds. _J Wound Care_ **15**(8): 344–6

Lofty M, Badra G, Burham W, Alenzi FQ (2006) Combined use of honey, bee propolis and myrrh on healing a deep, infected wound in a patient with diabetes mellitus. _Br J Biomed Sci_ **63**(4): 171–3

Maeda Y, Loughrey A, Philip Earle JA, _et al_ (2008) Antibacterial activity of honey against community-associated methicillin-resistant _Staphylococcus aureus_ (CA-MRSA). _Complementary Ther Clin Pract_ **14**: 77–82

Marshall C (2004) The ankle:brachial pressure index. A critical appraisal. _Br J Podiatry_ **7**(4): 93–5

McInnes A, White R (2007) The diabetic foot. In: Lindsay E, White R, eds. _Leg Ulcers and Problems of the Lower Limb: An holistic approach_. Wounds UK, Aberdeen: 189–206

McIntosh C, Newton V (2005) Superficial Diabetic Foot Ulcers. In: White R, ed. _Skin Care in Wound Management: Assessment, prevention and treatment_. Wounds UK, Aberdeen: 47–73

McIntosh C (2007) Diabetic foot disease: An overview of current management strategies. National Association of Primary Care: _Diabetes Supplement Summer 2007_: 4–11

McIntosh C, Newton V (2007) Diabetic foot ulcers. In: Ousey K, McIntosh C, eds. _Lower Extremity Wounds: A problem based approach_. John Wiley and Sons Publications, London

McIntosh C (2008) Healing wounds with honey. _Skills 4 Nurses_ **1**: 44–6

Molan P (2001) Honey as a topical antibacterial agent for treatment of infected wounds (online). Available online at: www.worldwidewounds.com/2001/november/Molan/honey-as-topical-agent.html [last accessed 02/09/08]

Molan PC, Betts JA (2004) Clinical usage of honey as a wound dressing: an update. _J Wound Care_ **13**(9): 353–6

National Institute for Health and Clinical Excellence (2004) _Clinical guidelines for Type 2 diabetes: Prevention and management of foot problems, clinical guideline 10_. NICE, London

Petrova NL, Moniz C, Elias DA (2007) Is there a systemic inflammatory response in the acute Charcot foot. _Diabetes Care_ **30**(4): 997–8

Plank J, Haas W, Rakovac I, _et al_ (2003) Evaluation of the impact of chiropodist care in the secondary prevention of foot ulcerations in diabetic subjects. _Diabetes Care_ **26**(6): 1691–5

Price PE (2008) Education, psychology and 'compliance'. *Diabetes Metab Res Rev* **24**: 101–5

Reiber GE, Vileikyte L, Boyko EJ, *et al* (1999) Causal pathways for incident lower-extremity ulcers in patients with diabetes from two settings. *Diabetes Care* **22**: 157–62

Ribu L, Hanestad BR, Moum T, *et al* (2007) A comparison of the health related quality of life in patients with diabetic foot ulcers, with a diabetes group and a non-diabetes group from the general population. *Qual Life Res* **16**(2): 179–89

Richard JL, Sotto A, Jourdan N, *et al* (2008) Risk factors and healing impact of multidrug-resistant bacteria in diabetic foot ulcers. *Diabetes Metab* **34**(4): 363–9

Ronnemaa T, Hamalainen H, Toikka T, *et al* (1997) Evaluation of the impact of podiatrist care in the primary prevention of foot problems in diabetic subjects. *Diabetes Care* **20**: 1833–7

Shaw JE, Boulton AJM (2001) The diabetic foot. In: Beard JD, Gaines PA, eds. *Vascular and Endovascular Surgery*. 2nd edn. WB Saunders, London: 105–26

Sheppard SJ (2005) Antibiotic treatment of infected diabetic foot ulcers. *J Wound Care* **14**(6): 260–3

Singh N, Armstrong DG, Lipsky BA (2005) Preventing foot ulcers in patients with diabetes. *JAMA* **293**: 217–28

Stanaway S, Johnson D, Moulik P, *et al* (2007) Methicillin-resistant *Staphyloccus aureus* (MRSA) isolation from diabetic foot ulcers correlates with nasal MRSA carriage. *Diabetes Res Clin Pract* **75**: 47–50

Tentolouris N, Jude EB, Smirnof E, *et al* (1999) Methicillin-resistant *Staphyloccus aureus*: an increasing problem in the diabetic foot clinic. *Diabetes Med* **16**: 767–71

UK Prospective Diabetes Study (UKPDS) (1998) Intensive blood-glucose control with sulphonylureas or insulin compared with conventional treatment and risk of complications in patients with type 2 diabetes. (UKPDS 33) *Lancet* **352**(9131): 837–53

Vandepuute J, van Waeyenberge PH (2003) Clinical investigation of L-Mesitran 'a honey based ointment'. *EWMA J* **3**(2): 8–11

van Schie CHM (2008) Neuropathy; mobility and quality of life. *Diabetes Metab Res Rev* **24**(Suppl 1): S45–S51

Vardi A, Barzilay Z, Linder N, *et al* (1998) Local application of honey for treatment of neonatal post-operative wound infections. *Acta Paediatr* **87**(4): 429–32

Vowden P (1999) Doppler ultrasound in the management of the diabetic foot. *Diabetic Foot* **2**(1): 16–17

Vowden K, Vowden P (2002) *Hand-held Doppler ultrasound: The assessment of lower limb arterial and venous disease*. (Suppl) Huntleigh Healthcare Ltd, Cardiff

Wadi M, Al-Amin H, Farouq A, Kashef H, Khaled SA (1987) Sudanese bee honey in the treatment of suppurated wounds. *Arab Medico* **3**: 1618

Wild S, Roglic G, Green A, *et al* (2004) Global prevalence of diabetes. *Diabetes Care* 27: 1047–53

Williams G, Pickup JC (1999) *Handbook of Diabetes*. 2nd edn. Blackwell Science, Oxford

Young MJ, Breddy JL, Veves A, *et al* (1994) The prediction of diabetic neuropathic foot ulceration using vibration perception thresholds. A prospective study. *Diabetes Care* 17(6): 557–60

Ziegler D (2008) Painful diabetic neuropathy: treatment and future aspects. *Diabetes Metab Res Rev* 24(Suppl 1): S52–S57

CHAPTER 9

EFFICACY OF HONEY AS A DEBRIDING AND pH MODULATING AGENT

Georgina Gethin

Honey has been used in wound healing for centuries for diabetic ulcers, Fournier's gangrene, animal bites, burns and scalds, venous ulcers, pressure ulcers, as well as other conditions. There is considerable variability in the type of honey used, its frequency of application and the condition of the wound bed to which it is applied. It is therefore important to understand how honey interacts with the wound bed and how this can effect wound healing. Of particular interest is how honey works to deslough the wound and its influence on wound pH.

Understanding slough

The removal of devitalised and/or necrotic tissue, slough and biofilm from a wound is essential to optimise healing when consistent with patient and treatment goals. Slough is a variant of necrotic tissue and is visible in the wound bed as moist, stringy, loose tissue, that is typically yellow in colour which represents a complex mixture of fibrin, deoxyribonucleo-protein, serous exudate, leucocytes and bacteria (Thomas *et al*, 1999). Slough is generated during the normal inflammatory phase when dead cells accumulate in exudate (Ayello and Cuddigan, 2004). Excessive deposition of slough is usually limited by surgical debridement, which is achieved by incoming leukocytes that remove devitalised tissue and foreign material. The body normally keeps pace with the build up of slough through a natural process of autolysis. Autolytic debridement of slough in the normal wound healing process is achieved through the phagocytic and enzymatic action of polymorphonuclear leukocytes (PMNs) and leucocytes (Ross and Odland, 1968).

Persistent necrotic tissue in the wound provides a suitable environment for bacterial proliferation and infection. The release of bacterial exotoxins helps to perpetuate the early inflammatory state and prevent progression towards healing (Himel, 1995). Additionally, some bacteria produce ammonia which, in itself, is necrotising and can impair oxygenation of the tissues by raising the wound pH (Leveen *et al*, 1973). The normal processes of wound repair include enzymatic mechanisms of 'damage repair' designed to remove wound detritus, including fibrin and necrotic material, prior to tissue regeneration. Some of the enzymes involved, matrix metalloproteinases (MMPs), are unregulated in chronic wounds and so exert a deleterious effect on healing through the continued degradation of extracellular matrix (Schultz *et al*, 2005). Continual breakdown of wound tissue is visible as slough in the wound.

Slough and necrotic tissue also cause wound hypoxia which inhibits development of granulation tissue and slows re-epithelisation (Konig *et al*, 2005). Furthermore, lymphocyte and macrophage migration is hampered in the presence of slough or necrotic tissue (Thomas and Fear, 1993; Morison and Moffatt, 1995).

Debridement is the removal of devitalised or infected tissue, fibrin, or foreign material ('debris') from a wound and is an important intervention that stimulates healing (Sieggreen and Maklebust, 1997; Gottrup, 1999; Falanga, 1999; National Institute for Health and Clinical Excellence [NICE], 2001; Steed *et al*, 2006). Debridement further assists in the reduction of levels of bacteria as it removes not only the bacteria, but the environment that supports their persistence. Methods of debridement include surgical, sharp, mechanical, enzymatic, biosurgical and autolytic. This chapter will review the role of honey in debridement and proposes that it contributes to autolytic debridement.

Autolytic debridement is dependent on the local wound environment, particularly in wound temperature, wound hydration, pH and availability of enzymatic co-factors (Ayello and Cuddigan, 2004). It is a highly selective method that requires minimal clinical training, is painless for the patient and eventually leaves a clearly demarcated line between viable and non-viable tissue (Sieggreen and Maklebust, 1997; Ayello and Cuddigan, 2004). One of its limitations is that older individuals produce decreased amounts of endogenous proteases, such as collagenase, in their wound fluid (Himel, 1995). This decreased production and activity of endogenous collagenase may lead to insufficient debridement of necrotic tissue, a reduction of granulation tissue and matrix remodelling, as well as less proliferation and migration of keratinocytes (Baharestani,

1999). A further disadvantage of autolytic debridement is that it is not recommended for clinically infected wounds, i.e. those with a high potential for anaerobic infection or if there is ischaemia (Baharestani, 1999; Ayello and Cuddigan, 2004; Davies, 2004).

Natural autolytic debridement occurs to some extent in all wounds. Here macrophages phagocytose bacteria and endogenous proteolytic enzymes, such as collagenase, elastase and myeloperoxidase, and they liquefy and spontaneously separate necrotic tissue and pseudoeschar from healthy tissue (Baharestani, 1999). Wound fluid contains macrophages, and neutrophils that digest and solubilise this necrotic tissue (Sieggreen and Malkebust, 1997).

Wound healing is thus delayed in the presence of slough and while many topical treatment options are available for its removal, to date, systematic reviews have concluded that no one agent has demonstrated superior efficacy over another and there are no studies which have compared the option of debriding with not debriding (Bradley *et al*, 1999; Lewis *et al*, 2001).

Clinical evidence of honey as a debriding agent

The physical nature of honey means that it acts intimately with the wound environment and has the ability to connect directly with all surfaces (Gethin and Cowman, 2005). This may enhance its wound management potential. Honey is a highly osmotic substance (Thomas, 1990; Cooper *et al*, 2001). Colloidal honey has a low osmotic pressure and when in contact with the wound goes through a physiological change (Seymore and West, 1951). The hygroscopic quality of honey permits its dilution by tissue fluids, so that the colloidal sugar molecules pass into solution, the osmotic pressure increases and plasmolysis of the tissue becomes more active (Seymore and West, 1951). The high osmolarity supports the outflow of fluid from deep wound tissue to the wound surface, thus aiding cleansing, debridement and reducing oedema (Thomas, 1990; Cooper *et al*, 2001). It has been argued that this osmotic pressure could possibly dehydrate delicate new cells on the wound surface and delay healing (Forrest, 1982). However, the flux of fluid from cells in the deep regions of a wound may rapidly replace fluid lost from the wound surface (Chirife *et al*, 1983) and prevent dehydration of the surface. This effect is described in more detail in *Chapter 2*.

Within the medical literature, many case studies of honey rapidly debriding a variety of both acute and chronic wounds in a timeframe of two days to three weeks have been recorded (Dunford, 2001; Kingsley, 2001; van der Weyden, 2003; Gray, 2005; Blaser et al, 2007). Large case series and pilot studies have also supported this effect. A pilot study using Honeysoft® (formerly Dermaprof, now Taureon, The Netherlands) reported on thirteen complex wounds of varying aetiologies which were effectively debrided with reduced exudate, malodour and improved epithelisation over three weeks (Ahmed et al, 2003). This rapid debridement was also achieved when a local Nigerian honey was used in the treatment of 43 cases of pyomyositis abscess in children (Okeniyi et al, 2005). Honey was applied daily in the latter study and the authors reported shorter duration of antibiotic use and hospital stay when honey was used, than in the EUSOL control.

In the management of Fournier's gangrene, three large case studies involving 111 patients reported rapid efficacy of honey in removing sloughy tissue and reducing exudate and malodour (Hejase et al, 1996; Subrahmanyam and Ugane, 2004; Tahmaz et al, 2006). In the latter three studies there was regional variation in the type of honey used, which included Indiana (USA), Turkey (Europe) and India. Twenty-five paediatric patients with superficial thermal burns of $< 50\%$ body area had no slough formation when a local (Indian) honey was used (Bangroo, 2005). Within all of these studies, a reduction in exudate and elimination of malodour was also reported. These studies support the premise that the high osmotic activity of honey contributes to wound debridement. As the pH of the honey was not stated in these studies, its contribution to the debridement process cannot be guaranteed.

The largest randomised controlled trial (RCT) of the use of manuka honey as a debriding agent was conducted in 108 cases of venous ulceration (Gethin and Cowman, 2008; Chapter 8). Venous ulcers with $\geq 50\%$ slough in the wound bed were randomised to either a manuka honey dressing (Woundcare 18+, Comvita New Zealand) or hydrogel therapy (IntraSite Gel®, Smith & Nephew, UK). Patients were excluded if infection was present or developed during the course of the study. Wounds were dressed weekly for four weeks and compression therapy continued in all cases. The mean percentage reduction in slough was 67% in the manuka honey group, versus 52.59% in the hydrogel group ($p < 0.054$). The mean area covered in slough reduced from 85–29% in those treated with honey, versus a reduction from 78–43% in those treated with hydrogel ($p < 0.065$). An important finding in the latter study was that wounds in which $> 50\%$ slough was removed by week 4 had a greater probability of healing at week 12 (CI 1.92, 9.7, RR 3.3, p0.029), thus supporting the expert opinion that removal of slough promotes healing (Gethin and Cowman, 2008). Collectively, these studies support the premise that honey contributes to wound debridement. As the pH of honey was not stated in some of these studies, its contribution to the debridement process cannot be assumed.

Understanding wound pH

The pH notation is a measurement of the concentration of H^+ in a solution (Soloman *et al*, 1990). Because a logarithmic scale is used for all pH measurements, actual acidity increases much faster than the numerical change in pH might seem to indicate (Ganong, 2001). A pH of 5 is 10 times more acidic than a pH of 6, that is, it represents a ten-fold increase in hydrogen ion concentration (Soloman *et al*, 1990).

The pH of human tissue is stabilised by the buffering capacity of the body fluid. A buffer is a solution of two or more chemical compounds that is capable of preventing a marked change in H^+ concentration when either an acid or base is added (Soloman *et al*, 1990). Buffers include blood and cell proteins. The protein buffering system is the most abundant buffering system in the blood and tissue cells. Proteins are able to take hydrogen ions out of solution and bind them to their structure, thereby decreasing the hydrogen ion concentration of the solution and minimising pH changes (Soloman *et al*, 1990). It is notable that fluid from chronic non-healing wounds has low total protein levels compared to serum, and that these levels increase as the wound heals (Stacy and Trengove, 2000; Timothy *et al*, 2000). Haemoglobin is an intracellular buffer so that when intracellular hydrogen ions are formed they are buffered by haemoglobin. When oxyhaemoglobin releases oxygen, the reduced haemoglobin possesses a net negative charge that can bind hydrogen ions (Soloman *et al*, 1990).

The surface pH of chronic wounds have been recorded within the range 7.15–8.9, representing both healing and non-healing states (Wilson *et al*, 1979; Romanelli *et al*, 1997). The pH of a wound was found to decrease during healing (Hoffman *et al*, 1999). Recording the surface pH over 24 weeks has shown that surface pH measurements move from alkaline to acidic levels as healing occurs (Roberts *et al*, 1997). Chronic wounds which maintain an elevated alkaline pH have demonstrated lower rates of healing compared to those in which the pH is closer to neutral (Roberts *et al*, 1997; Gethin *et al*, 2008). This is also the case in acute wounds in which the failure of split-thickness skin grafts to heal was correlated with an alkaline pH (Leveen _et al_, 1973).

Surface pH is not influenced by the depth of the wound, but rather by the presence of various tissue types. In pressure ulcers, the pH of the wound was lower in the presence of epithelial tissue (Tsukada _et al_, 1992). The pH of stage 1 pressure ulcers was similar to that of intact skin (range 5.4–5.6), but increased to 6.9 for stage 2 and 7.6 for stage 3 pressure ulcers (Tsukada _et al_, 1992). Wounds in which epithelial tissue was evident had a mean pH of 6.0, compared to a mean of 7.8 for wounds with no epithelial tissue ($p < 0.001$). The presence of necrotic and devitalised tissue in the wound causes an increased metabolic load on the wound resulting in tissue hypoxia and an elevated alkaline pH (Gethin _et al_, 2008), of which there are many potential causes. Excessive breakdown of the extracellular matrix (ECM), and consequently the wound itself, occurs more readily in an alkaline environment (Greener _et al_, 2005; Gethin _et al_, 2008).

This alkaline environment helps to perpetuate the non-healing state via the action of proteases. MMPs are a family of more than 20 proteases that collectively can degrade most of the components of the ECM (Greener _et al_, 2005). They are enzymes that have the ability to cleave proteins at optimal pH values above 5.0. This ability is referred to as the 'activity' of the proteases and is dependent on both the amount of proteases present and on the presence of inhibitors (Hoffman _et al_, 1999). Every protease has peak enzyme activity at certain pH levels, where the protein is broken down more rapidly than at other pH values (Greener _et al_, 2005).

In vitro chronic wound fluid analysis showed Cathepsin G to have peak activity at pH 7.0, and each of elastase, plasmin and MMP-2 at pH 8.0 (Greener _et al_, 2005). In addition, human neutrophil elastase was found to be particularly pH dependent with maximal observed activity at pH 8.3 (Greener _et al_, 2005). Elastase contributes to the proteolytic activity of non-healing wounds, and excess elastase at the wound bed can cause endothelial damage, as well as degradation of the epidermal/ dermal junction. Additionally, proteases are not only produced by the wound itself, but also by bacteria. This is important as chronic wounds can harbour at least four different types of bacteria at any one time and, indeed, the bacterial flora may change over time (Trengove _et al_, 1996; Bowler 1998).

As with all physiological processes, wound healing is dependent on an adequate supply of oxygen (Hunt and Beckert, 2005). Oxygen delivery to a particular tissue depends not only on the amount of O_2 entering the lungs, but also the adequacy of pulmonary gas exchange, the blood flow to the tissue and the capacity of the blood to carry oxygen (Ganong, 2001). Additionally, oxygen delivery to damaged tissue, particularly in the chronic wound, is dependent both on perfusion and diffusion (Hunt and Beckert, 2005). A lowering of pH (more acidic) by 0.6 releases almost 50% more oxygen and a five-fold increase in release of oxygen by a shift of 0.9 pH units (Leveen *et al*, 1973). Within the chronic wound this may be significant, as the likelihood of healing is high if tissue oxygen tension (pO2) is >40 mmHg, but healing is unlikely to occur at levels of <20 mmHg (Hunt and Beckert, 2005). In chronic recurrent wounds, particularly venous leg ulcers, the skin and local vasculature become scarred and atrophic, thus raising permanent obstacles to the transport of oxygen (Hunt and Beckert, 2005).

Other effects of lowering the pH to a more acidic environment include:

- reducing the toxicity of bacterial end-products such as ammonia
- decreasing protease activity
- enhancing the destruction of abnormal collagen in the ulcer bed
- increasing macrophage and fibroblast activity
- promoting angiogenesis
- controlling enzyme activity (Romanelli *et al*, 1997; Molan, 2002; Brett, 2003; Greener *et al*, 2005).

Some wound dressings can contribute to lowering the wound pH. The permeability of dressings to carbon dioxide is important, as surface wounds may develop a respiratory alkalosis as a result of the loss of carbon dioxide into the air (Thomas, 1990). Thus, occlusion of the wound prevents the loss of carbon dioxide and consequently prevents the wound from entering an alkaline state. Honey may be particularly useful as a pH modulating agent due to its low pH of 3.5–4.5.

Honey as a pH modulating agent

The pH of honey from European honeybees (*Apis mellifera*) is in the range of 3.5–4.5. Some geographical regions such as Pakistan have honeys with a reported pH range of up to 6.3 (Kamal *et al*, 2002). When undiluted, the acidity of honey is a significant antibacterial factor. The acidity of honey may assist in the antibacterial action of neutrophils, as the pH inside the phagocytic vacuole that is involved in killing ingested bacteria is acidic (Molan, 1998).

The efficacy of manuka honey as a pH modulating agent has been investigated (Gethin *et al*, 2008). In this study, 20 patients with chronic non-healing wounds were treated with manuka honey dressings (Apinate, Comvita New Zealand) over a two-week period. Wound size and pH in all patients was measured at the start of the study and clinical evaluation of the wound bed was made; observations were repeated after two weeks. Mean pH reduced from 7.72 (SD 0.33) to 7.26 (SD 0.53) ($p < 0.001$). Wounds with a pH ≤7.50 ($n = 4$) and ≤7.60 ($n = 6$) at the start had a 39% and 30% reduction in size respectively at two weeks. Importantly, this study demonstrated that a reduction of 0.1 pH units was correlated with an 8.1% reduction size ($p 0.012$). Clinical evaluation of the wounds with slough showed that a decrease in slough was associated with a 29% decrease in wound size and a mean pH at the start of 7.6. The pH of the honey dressing was 3.5. This would support the premise that the pH modulating effect of manuka honey contributes to the desloughing effect.

While it has been shown that healing takes place in an acid environment, one study using an ointment made from natural royal jelly and panthenol with a pH of 7.5, suggested that healing was promoted by the creation of an alkaline environment (Abdelatif *et al*, 2008). In this study, sixty patients with limb-threatening diabetic foot ulcers were treated. After six months all of the patients with a Wagner scale 1 ulcer ($n = 26$) had healed, 92% of the patients with a Wagner scale 2 ulcer ($n = 22$) had healed, and all of the patients with a Wagner scale 3 ulcer ($n = 10$) had healed. The authors commented that the tight glycaemic control offered to all patients within the study would have positively influenced wound healing. However, the premise that healing was enhanced by the creation of an alkaline environment warrants further study, as the study group was specific to diabetic foot ulcers and is thus not generalisable to other wound aetiologies.

Conclusion

In the hierarchy of evidence, honey, in particular manuka honey, has demonstrated efficacy as a debriding agent in case studies, case series and RCTs. This effect is due to its osmotic action, antibacterial action and pH modulation, each of which work to modulate the environment which favours slough production initially and its consequent removal. Honey can thus be considered to act as an autolytic debriding agent.

References

Abdelatif M, Yakoot M, Etmaan M (2008) Safety and efficacy of a new honey ointment on diabetic foot ulcers: a prospective pilot study. *J Wound Care* 17(3): 108–10

Ahmed A, Hoekstra M, Hage J, Karim R (2003) Honey-medicated dressing: transformation of an ancient remedy into modern therapy. *Ann Plastic Surg* 50(2): 143–8

Ayello E, Cuddigan J (2004) Debridment: controlling the necrotic/cellular burden. *Adv Skin Wound Care* 17(2): 66–75

Baharestani M (1999) *The Clinical Relevance of Debridement*. Springer-Verlag, Heidelberg

Bangroo AK (2005) Honey dressing in paediatric burns. *J Indian Assoc Paediatr Surgeons* 10(3): 172–5

Blaser G, Santos K, Bode U, Vetter H, Simon A (2007) Effect of medical honey on wounds colonised or infected with MRSA. *J Wound Care* 1(3): 325–8

Brett D (2003) Wound pH. In: Brett D, ed. *A historic review of topical enzymatic debridement*. McMahon publishing, New York: 4–90

Bradley M, Cullum N, Sheldon T (1999b) The debridement of chronic wounds: A systematic review. *Health Technology Assessment* 3(17 Pt 1)

Chirife J, Herszage L, Joseph A, Kohn E (1983) *In vitro* study of bacterial growth inhibition in concentrated sugar solutions; microbiological basis for the use of sugar in treating infected wounds. *Antimicrob Agents Chemother* 23(5): 766–73

Cooper R, Molan P, Krishnamoorthy L, Harding K (2001) Manuka honey used to heal a recalcitrant surgical wound. *Eur J Clin Microbiol Infect Dis* 20: 758–9

Davies P (2004) Current thinking on the management of necrotic and sloughy wounds. *Prof Nurse* 19(10): 34–6

Dunford C (2001) Treatment of wound infection in a patient with mantle cell lymphoma. *Br J Nurs* 10(16): 1058–65

Falanga V (2002) The clinical relevance of wound bed preparation. In: Falanga V, Harding K, eds. *The Clinical Relevance of Debridement*. Springer-Verlag, Heidelberg

Forrest R (1982) Early history of wound treatment. *J Roy Soc Med* 75: 198–205

Ganong WF (2001) *Review of Medical Physiology*. McGraw-Hill Medical Publishing, New York

Gethin G, Cowman S (2005) Case series of use of Manuka honey in leg ulceration. *Int Wound J* 2(1): 10–15

Gethin G, Cowman S (2008) Manuka honey vs hydrogel, a prospective, open label, multicentre randomised controlled trial to compare desloughing efficacy and healing outcomes in venous ulcers. *J Clin Nurs* Aug 23. [Epub ahead of print]

Gethin G, Cowman S, Conroy R (2008) The impact of Manuka honey dressings on surface pH of chronic wounds. *Int Wound J* 5(2): 185–95

Gottrup F (1999) Preface. In: Falanga V, Harding K, eds. *The Clinical Relevance of Debridement*. Springer-Verlag, Heidelberg

Gray D (2005) Mesitran Ointment Case Studies. *Wounds UK* Supplement, 1(3): S32–35

Greener B, Hughes A, Bannister N, Douglass J (2005) Proteases and pH in chronic wounds. *J Wound Care* 14(2): 59–61

Hejase MJ, Simonin JE, Bihrle R, Coogan CL (1996) Genital Fournier's gangrene: experience with 38 patients. *Urology* 47(5): 734–9

Himel H (1995) Wound Healing: focus on the chronic wound. *Wounds* Suppl A(5): 70–7

Hoffman R, Noble J, Eagle M (1999) The use of proteases as prognostic markers for the healing of venous leg ulcers. *J Wound Care* 8(6): 272–6

Hunt TK, Beckert S (2005) Therapeutical and practical aspects of oxygen in wound healing. In: Lee B, ed. *The Wound Management Manual*. McGraw-Hill Medical, USA

Kamal A, Raza S, Rashid N, Hameed T, Gilani M, Qureshi A, Nasim K (2002) Comparative study of honey collected form different flora of Pakistan. *OnLine Journal of Biological Sciences* 2(9): 626–7

Kingsley A (2001) The use of honey in the treatment of infected wounds: case studies. *Br J Nurs* 10(22) Tissue Viability Supplement: S13–14

Konig M, Vanscheidt W, Augustin M, Kapp H (2005) Enzymatic versus autolytic debridement of chronic leg ulcers: a prospective randomized trial. *J Wound Care* 14(7): 320–3

Leveen H, Falk G, Borek B, Diaz C, Lynfield Y, Wynkoop B, *et al* (1973) Chemical acidification of wounds. An adjuvant to healing and the unfavourable action of alkalinity and ammonia. *Ann Surg* 178(6): 745–50

Lewis R, Whiting P, ter Riet G, O'Meara S, Glanville J (2001) A rapid and systematic review of the clinical effectiveness and cost-effectiveness of debriding agents in treating surgical wounds healing by secondary intention. *Health Technology Assessment* 5(14)

Molan P (1998) A brief review of the use of honey as a clinical dressing. *Primary Intention* 6(4): 148–58

Molan P (2002) Re-introducing honey in the management of wounds and ulcers — theory and practice. *Ostomy/Wound Management* 48(11): 28–40

Morison M, Moffatt C (1995) *A Colour Guide to the Assessment and Management of Leg Ulcers*. Mosby, Aylesbury: 130

National Institute for Health and Clinical Excellence (2001) Guidance on the use of debriding agents and specialist wound care clinics for difficult to heal surgical wounds. Technology Appraisal Guidance No 24. NICE, London

Okeniyi J, Olubanjo O, Ogunlesi T, Oyelami O (2005) Comparison of healing in incised abscess wounds with honey and EUSOL dressing. *J Altern Complement Med* 11(3): 511–13

Roberts G, Hammad L, Creevy J, Shearman C, Mani R (1997) Physical changes in dermal tissues around chronic venous ulcers. In 7th European Conference on advances in wound management. Journal of European Wound Management Association, Harrogate, UK: 104–105

Romanelli M, Schipani E, Piaggesi A, Barachini P (1997) *Evaluation of surface pH of venous leg ulcers under Allevyn dressings.* The Royal Society of Medicine Press, London

Ross R, Odland G (1968) Human wound repair II: Inflammatory cells, epithelial-mesenchymal interrelations, and fibrogenesis. *J Cell Biol* 39(1): 152–68

Schultz G, Mozingo D, Romanelli M, Claxton K (2005) Wound healing and TIME: new concepts and scientific applications. *Wound Rep Regen* 13(4): S1–S11

Seymore F, West F (1951) Honey — its role in medicine. *Med Times* 79(2): 104–7

Sieggreen M, Maklebust J (1997) Debridement: choices and challenges. *Adv Wound Care* 10(2): 32–7

Solomon E, Schmidt R, Adragna P (1990) *Human Anatomy and Physiology.* Saunders, USA

Stacy M, Trengove N (2000) Biochemical measurements of tissue and wound fluids. In: *Chronic Wound Healing.* WB Saunders, London

Steed DL, Hill DP, Woodske ME, Payne WG, Robson MC (2006) Wound-healing trajectories as outcome measures of venous stasis ulcer treatment. *Int Wound J* 3(1): 40–7

Subrahmanyam M, Ugane SP (2004) Honey dressing beneficial in treatment of Fournier's gangrene. *Indian J Surg* 66(2): 75–7

Thomas AM, Harding KG, Moore K (1999) The structure and composition of chronic wound eschar. *J Wound Care* 8(6): 285–7

Tahmaz L, Erdemir F, Kibar Y, Cosar A, Yalcyn O (2006) Fournier's gangrene: Report of thirty-three cases and a review of the literature. *Int J Urol* 13: 960–7

Thomas S (1990) Functions of a wound dressing. In: *Wound Management and Dressings.* The Pharmaceutical Press, London

Thomas S, Fear M (1993) Comparing two dressings for wound debridement. *J Wound Care* 2(5): 272–4

Timothy J, Hughes M, Cherry G, Taylor R (2000) Simple biochemical markers to assess chronic wounds. *Wound Rep Regen* 8(4): 264–9

Tonks A, Cooper RA, Price AJ, Molan PC, Jones KP (2001) Stimulation of TNF-alpha release in monocytes by honey. *Cytokine* 14(4): 240–2

Trengove N, Stacy M, Maculey S, Bennett N, Gibson J, Burslem F, *et al* (1999) Analysis of the acute and chronic wound environments: the role of proteases and their inhibitors. *Wound Rep Regen* 7: 442–52

Tsukada K, Tokunaga K, Iwama T, Mishima Y (1992) The pH changes of pressure ulcers related to the healing process of wounds. *Wounds: a compendium of clinical research and practice* 4(1): 16–20

van der Weyden EA (2003) The use of honey for the treatment of two patients with pressure ulcers. *Br J Community Nurs* 8(12): S14–20

Wilson M, Henry M, Quill R, Byrne P (1979) The pH of varicose ulcer surfaces and its relationship to healing. *VASA* 8: 339–42

Chapter 10

Leg ulcers and honey: a review of recent controlled studies

Laura Bolton

Venous ulcers (VU) are the most common chronic leg ulcers in the ambulatory elderly, afflicting an estimated 0.2–1% of the total population. Prevalence increases with age to 1–3% of those over 60 years of age at any given time (Margolis *et al*, 2002). VU are severe clinical manifestations of chronic venous insufficiency (CVI), accounting for 60–70% of chronic ulcers of the lower limb (Mekkes *et al*, 2003; Abbade *et al*, 2005). A VU profoundly decreases a person's quality of life (QoL) (Cornwall 1986; Heit *et al*, 2001), causing social isolation (Margolis *et al*, 2002) and necessitating medical care and lost work time (Abbade *et al*, 2005; Luciana *et al*, 2005). VU occur on average about 13 years after the onset of CVI and recur after healing in 54–78% of patients (Cornwall *et al*, 1986; Phillips *et al*, 1994). It has been reported that VU are more prevalent in individuals with less economic resources and fewer years of education (Luciana *et al*, 2005).

Even most VU of long duration will heal during 12 weeks (Lyon *et al*, 1998) of consistent management with graduated, high (35 mmHg at the ankle decreasing to 10–15 mmHg at the infrapatellar notch) multi-layer elastic compression (Cullum *et al*, 2001), sustained for the full time it is worn and combined with appropriate local wound care. Optimal wound care includes a physiologically moist environment for healing (Leach, 2004) and, if needed to manage excess wound fluid, absorbent primary dressings such as alginate (Wipke-Tevis and Sae-Sia, 2005), or other absorbent dressings that minimise damage to the VU on removal. A dry VU may need a primary amorphous hydrogel to facilitate autolytic debridement (Romanelli, 1997). Surrounding venous dermatitis is typically managed with non-sensitising topical agents (Leach, 2004).

Patients can improve outcomes by actively participating in VU care, for example, by avoiding scratching or other trauma to the VU or surrounding skin, improving nutrition, e.g. avoiding salt and other foods that increase oedema, or stopping use of nicotine or other agents which restrict circulation. Patients and caregivers trained to recognise and report early signs of deterioration or infection such as unusual inflammation are valuable allies in averting serious VU complications. In addition to adhering to the prescribed lower leg compression, wound dressing and skin management regimens, patients help to improve their outcomes by regularly engaging in activities that reduce lower leg oedema, such as walking or ankle flexes sufficient to contract the calf muscle, or lower leg elevation above the heart periodically throughout the day until oedema recedes.

Despite such knowledge, VU remain slow and difficult to heal with annual VU management costs estimated at £200 million in the United Kingdom, US$1 billion the United States (Mekkes *et al*, 2003), and $AU550–650 million in Australia. Each VU costs an estimated US$27,500 (Mekkes *et al*, 2003) to heal, with monthly home care costs estimated at US$2,500. Therapy that could speed healing would significantly improve VU patient quality of life, while reducing the clinical, social and economic burden of VU worldwide.

Topically applied honey has been explored as one option to foster wound healing. For example, pure natural honey covered with sterile gauze is reportedly superior to similarly covered silver sulfadiazine in healing, reducing bacterial burden and relieving pain of second-degree burns (Mashmood *et al*, 2006) and preventing radiation-induced mucositis in cancer patients (Motallebnejad *et al*, 2008). Honey effects vary with floral source, geographic location and post-harvesting processing conditions. In addition to the typical sources of clinical wound care variability, this adds to the difficulty of interpreting its clinical efficacy and safety on wounds. Despite this variability, a recent review (Molan, 2006) concluded that there is growing evidence for honey in improving healing rates, reducing pain or damage on dressing removal and decreasing wound bacteria, necrotic tissue, malodour, inflammation, oedema, exudate and scarring, suggesting that clinical decisions weigh the evidence for honey against that for other topical wound care modalities (Molan, 2006). To simplify decisions for clinicians considering using topical honey to manage leg ulcers, we summarise recent controlled studies exploring relative safety and/or efficacy of honey on leg ulcers.

Methods

Articles found in the MEDLINE or Cochrane databases including the combination of terms 'honey, leg ulcer, controlled' and related derivative references found by searching Google or by contacting authors were reviewed for comparative safety and efficacy on any measured leg ulcer outcome. Evidence criteria used to support conclusions (*Table 10.1*) included at least two clinically relevant VU randomised controlled trials (RCT) or a systematic review or meta-analysis, including at least two RCTs (Registered Nurses Association of Ontario [RNAO], 2005; Wound, Ostomy and Continence Nurses Society [WOCN], 2008), and case studies or opinion as the lowest level of evidence.

Table 10.1: Evidence criteria used to evaluate support of honey effects on venous ulcer outcome	
Level A	Results of two or more randomised controlled trials (RCTs) in leg ulcer patients providing support for efficacy
Level B	Results of one leg ulcer RCT, plus one or more historically controlled or non-randomised controlled leg ulcer study providing support
Level C	This rating requires one or more of the following: • C1: Results of one controlled trial, eg. RCT or non-randomised or historically controlled trial • C2: Results of at least two case series (CS) or descriptive studies or a cohort study in humans • C3: Expert opinion (EO)

Results

Healing effects

RCT evidence supporting topical honey in the management of leg ulcers is presented in *Table 10.2*. The highest level of evidence supported manuka honey made from nectar of the *Leptospermum scoparium* bush found in New Zealand and Australia. This consisted of two RCTs (Jull *et al*, 2008; Gethin, 2008) on a total of 241 venous leg ulcers treated with manuka honey, plus 43 leg ulcers (*Table 10.3*) of varying aetiology on 40 patients also managed with manuka honey in an historically controlled trial (Dunford and Hanano, 2004), and a case-controlled study of similar leg ulcers on the same patient (*n*=3) (Milne, 2008). In the first RCT, Jull *et al* (2008) compared healing outcomes of relatively small, short-duration VU managed with multi-layer compression and either a calcium alginate dressing impregnated with manuka honey ($n=187$), or primary dressings according to 'usual care' ($n=181$). Dressings and compression were changed 'as needed'. Complete healing occurred in 12 weeks in 55.6% of the manuka honey group and 49.7% of the 'usual care' group ($p=0.258$). Findings were similar after adjusting for ulcer duration, size and study centre. The second manuka honey RCT (Gethin, 2008) used a primary hydrocellular foam dressing impregnated with either manuka honey ($n=54$), or an amorphous hydrogel ($n=54$) on longer duration VU covered with at least 50% slough. Subjects studied by Gethin (2008) had larger VU than those studied by Jull *et al* (2008). Both dressings were applied once-weekly for four weeks in conjunction with up to four layers of compression bandaging. After this time, follow-on treatment varied between patients based on local investigators' clinical assessments. Patients treated with manuka honey in the second study showed earlier epithelisation ($p=0.042$) and a greater percent of patients healed at 12 weeks ($p=0.037$) compared to hydrogel controls. The percent of patients healed at 12 weeks remained more for the manuka honey group ($p=0.025$) after using Margolis (2000) standardised scores to adjust for VU area $>5\,cm^2$ and duration >6 months, two risk factors for delayed VU healing.

Based on these studies, B level evidence (one RCT plus two quasi-experimental case series) supports the healing benefit of manuka honey on venous leg ulcers when applied within a protocol using topical manuka honey as the primary modality in contact with the leg ulcer covered with a foam, contact layer or calcium alginate dressing, and used with multilayer compression bandages to aid venous return when indicated.

Natural, non-manuka honey was studied in a non-randomised controlled study (*Table 10.3*) on 38 patients whose 50 non-venous, non-diabetic, post-traumatic or post-infected non-malignant leg ulcers were treated topically for four weeks with undiluted unprocessed honey, compared to the same honey plus phenytoin paste or phenytoin paste alone (Oluwatosin *et al*, 2000). All modalities were covered with sterile gauze. The only significant differences reported were a transient increase in percent area reduction for phenytoin paste without honey, which did not continue after the first week of the study, and a decrease in leg ulcer area of more mm^2 during week four for the other two groups of patients. At this time, there is currently insufficient evidence to support a healing benefit from the use of pure natural honey not from the *Leptospermum scoparium* bush on post-traumatic or post-infected leg ulcers.

Safety

The most frequent adverse events reported in the manuka honey RCTs were VU pain of unrecorded intensity, deterioration of the VU or surrounding skin, and infection. These are occasional characteristics of VU and not clearly associated with honey. No episodes of pain were reported in the RCT applying a foam dressing impregnated with either manuka honey or hydrogel to VU of median 9.9 or 10.5 cm^2 areas respectively (Gethin, 2008). In contrast, the RCT applying an alginate dressing impregnated with manuka honey to smaller VU (median area 2.7 cm^2) (Jull _et al_, 2008) reported frequent VU pain in the alginate-manuka honey group, although it was not possible to separate the effects of manuka honey from its simultaneously-applied alginate carrier dressing. In this study, 25% of manuka honey-alginate-treated subjects and 10% of 'usual care' patients reported one or more episodes of pain as an adverse event ($p < 0.001$), 'but only four participants (2.1%) gave pain as the reason for withdrawing from treatment, suggesting that the pain was short-lived or tolerable'.

Overall, 10 (3.0%) of 328 leg ulcer patients managed with any form of honey withdrew from studies due to pain. In the controlled studies using manuka honey (_Table 10.2_), four of more than 241 subjects (1.6%) gave pain as the reason for study withdrawal. In the historically controlled study, six of 40 patients with leg ulcers (15%) withdrew due to pain not necessarily related to the wound treatment, as more pain was associated with larger wound size or slower healing (Dunford and Hanano, 2004). Among up to 38 subjects treated with honey of unspecified origin in _Table 10.3_, no significant pain differences were reported between groups receiving or not receiving honey as leg ulcer treatment. No or decreasing pain tended to signal progressive healing (Dunford and Hanano, 2004). Increasing wound pain, an important sign of potential infection, was associated with delayed healing (Dunford and Hanano, 2004), as would be expected in any chronic or acute wound managed with any modality.

In the historically controlled study of 40 recalcitrant VU (Dunford and Hanano, 2004) dressed with a manuka honey-impregnated low-adherent sterile contact layer covered with a sterile dressing pad, patient-reported pain rated on a 1–5 scale decreased from 1.6 at baseline to 1.08 at study end, ($p < 0.02$ paired t-test or $p < 0.001$ for the mean of all 40 patients). Six patients complained of 'transient stinging pain' after applying the low-adherent layer laden with manuka honey, but this was never a reason for withdrawal. Pain

Table 10.2: RCTs supporting safety and/or efficacy of honey as a topical wound dressing on chronic leg ulcers

Reference (enrolment criteria)[1]	Patients enrolled		Study design	Clinical outcomes measured	Significant results (p>0.05)	
	Honey source (n) (dressing compression)	Control (n) (dressing compression)			Primary outcomes (p value honey versus control)	Other outcomes
Gethin et al, 2008 (patients >18 years of age with ABI ≥0.8 and a VU of area <100 cm² with ulcer bed >50% covered with slough	Manuka honey[1] (MH) 5 g/20cm² applied once per week (n=54) (hydrocellular foam, mostly 4-layer bandage) Baseline: mean duration MH 39.5 week; HG 29.9 week; area MH 10.5 cm², HG 9.9 cm²	Hydrogel (HG) 3g/20 cm² applied once per week (n=54) (hydrocellular foam, mostly 4-layer bandage)	Prospective M OL RCT with treatment lasting 4 weeks after which treatment varied per investigator	Primary: week 1–4 percentage of patients with leg ulcers covered with slough; week 12, percentage of patients with healed ulcers. Secondary: decrease in wound size; epithelisation; safety as adverse events (AEs)	At 12 weeks, 44% of MH and 33% of HG patients healed (0.037). At 4 weeks, MH had 67% slough decrease and HG 53% (0.054). Epithelisation was visible earlier for MH (0.042). Median wound size decreased from baseline to week 4 by 34% for MH, or 13% for HG (0.001)	No AEs were attributable to either treatment. Time to infection-related withdrawal was longer with MH (p<0.07); >50% 4-week slough reduction was associated with a higher probability of 12–week healing for all patients (0.029) Too few withdrew in MH (n=9), HG (n=17) for meaningful analysis
Jull et al, 2007 (patients >18 years of age with ABI >0.7 and a VU or VI AU able to tolerate compression) Baseline: mean duration MH 20 weeks, UC 16 weeks; mean area MH 2.7 cm², UC 2.6 cm²	Randomisation stratified by study centre and Margolis index. honey–calcium alginate dressing[2] changed with compression as clinically needed (n=187)	Usual care (UC) per nurse cnoice (n=181) (dressings included alginate, Hydrofiber®, hydrocolloid, foam, hydrogel or impregnated dressings) with compression as clinically needed (n=181)	Prospective M OL RCT with treatments given for 12 weeks, administered during compression changes	Primary: percent of participants completely healed at 12 weeks Other: heal time; ulcer area change from baseline, AEs, infections, health-related quality of life, (HRQL) cost-effectiveness	12 week healing: 104 (55%) of MH ulcers and 90 (49.7%) of UC ulcers (0.258). Mean time to heal 63.5 days for MH and 65.3 days for UC. (0.451). Findings similar adjusted for stratification variables	Clinical infection incidence 17.1% MH and 22.1% UC (0.228). More reports of pain in MH group (0.013) but intensity was not recorded. NS difference between groups in HRQL MH was slightly more cost-effective (NS) due to fewer hospitalised days (10 compared to 40 for UC group)

1 Woundcare 18+ (Comvita New Zealand, Ltd. Te Puke, New Zealand)

2 ApiNate™ UMF 12+; Comvita New Zeland Te Puke, New Zealand*

Key:

ABI	=	ankle brachial systolic blood pressure
AE	=	adverse event
CAD	=	calcium alginate dressing
HCAD	=	manuka honey in calcium alginate dressing
HRQL	=	health-related quality of life
hydrogel	=	HG
M	=	multicentre study
MH	=	manuka honey
NS	=	not statistically significant
OL	=	open label study
RCT	=	randomised clinical trial
UC	=	usual care
V/AU	=	mixed venous-arterial ulcer
VU	=	venous ulcer

*These calcium-alginate dressings impregnated with active _Leptospermum_ honey are now marketed as Medihoney brand Absorbent Calcium Alginate Dressing with _Leptospermum_ Honey (Derma Sciences, Inc. Princeton, New Jersey, USA)

Table 10.3: Controlled case series supporting safety and/or effects of honey as a topical wound dressing on chronic leg ulcers

Reference (enrolment criteria)	Patients enrolled		Study design M=multicentre OL=open label	Clinical outcomes measured wk=week	Significant results (p≤0.05; NS p>0.05)	
	Honey source (n) (dressing compression)	Control (n) (dressing compression)			Primary outcomes (p value honey versus control)	Other outcomes
Dunford and Hanano, 2004 (patients over 40 years of age with uninfected 35 VU, 2 AU or 3 V/AU with mean area 9.7 cm² <2 years duration, non-healing after 12 weeks despite compression and guideline-based care)	MH (40) applied for 12 weeks to a depth of 3 mm on a low-adherent, sterile wound contact layer (20 g per 10 x 10 cm) with a sterile dressing pad, under compression	Historic control (the same 40 patients) treatments included the same professionally applied compression to be used with MH after cross-over	Prospective OL 4-centre cross-over study. All aspects of care continued for 12 more weeks except to replace prior prescribed primary dressing with the MH dressing. All measures assessed every 2 weeks	Ulcer area, pain (McGill score), odour, satisfaction with current dressing regimen, leakage between dressing changes; skin problems, withdrawals, adverse events (AEs)	Mean pain scores for all 40 patients declined during study (0.001). 26 patients reporting odour said it decreased by the first assessment (0.001). Total mean wound area decreased on study (0.002) and 7 (17.5%) of the 40 patients healed. Patient satisfaction was high and correlated with above outcomes	Patients with initially larger wounds experienced more pain, slower healing and were more likely to withdraw (n = 13; 32.5%) from the study. 6 patients withdrew due to pain. None withdrew due to an adverse event. Healing was associated with declining ulcer pain, but not with dressing change frequency. Exudate declined with healing
Milne (2008) Patients with multiple leg ulcers comparable in size and non-viable tissue	MH (3) in calcium alginate dressing (HCAD)	Calcium alginate dressing (CAD) without honey (3)	Prospective OL single-centre 4-8-week study using each of two similar leg ulcers as a same-patient control	Autolytic debridement measured as % of non-viable tissue and decreases in wound area	Patient 1 returned to work at week 5 after HCAD-dressed ulcer closed 31%; CAD 18%. Patient 2 HCAD-dressed ulcer healed week 4, CAD week 8. Patient 3 HCAD ulcer healed by week 3. CAD ulcer healed 4 weeks after changed to HCAD	Ulcers resulted from pyoderma gangrenosum (patients 1 and 3), or scleroderma (patient 2)

Table 10.3: Cont.

Reference (enrolment criteria)	Patients enrolled		Study design M=multicentre O=open label	Clinical outcomes measured wk=week	Significant results (p≤0.05; NS p>0.05)	
	Honey source (N) (dressing compression)	Control (N) (dressing compression)			Primary outcomes (p value honey versus control)	Other outcomes
Oluwatosin, 2000 (38 out-patients with non-venous, non-diabetic leg ulcers of >6 week duration: mean 36.5 months)	Source not specified (number of patients or ulcers unclear in honey and mixture: honey+phenytoin groups) (no compression)	Phenytoin (22 ulcers) (no compression described in any patient in any group. Ulcers were not associated with venous insufficiency)	Prospective OL 4-week non-randomised controlled study of patients with post-traumatic or post-infective, non-malignant ulcers	1-4-wk healing rate/week (mm^2) and % area reduction; clinical ulcer status (0-9 scale); 4-week pain reduction from baseline (0-10 scale)	At baseline mean area was $33.4 cm^2$. More mm^2 of healing (p=0.04) occurred in ulcers receiving mixture (85) or honey (45) >phenytoin (-19) at 4 weeks. Phenytoin subjects had greater % reduction in area than that of other groups in week 1 (p=0.02)	Though there were no further significant differences, the best initial improvement in clinical score occurred in honey group (p=0.09). The only 4 ulcers that healed were in the phenytoin group (p=0.33 for week 4 clinical score)

Key:

AE	=	adverse event
CAD	=	calcium alginate dressing
HCAD	=	Manuka honey in calcium alginate dressing
MH	=	Manuka honey
V/AU	=	mixed venous-arterial ulcer
VU	=	venous ulcer

score fluctuations and intrinsic factors prevented a direct association of the pain with manuka honey. Pain was not reported when honey was used to manage leg ulcers associated with *pyoderma gangrenosum* or *scleroderma* (Milne, 2008), or as an adjunct to reduce the risk of split-thickness skin graft failure in six patients with an impaired blood supply to the VU receiving the graft (Schumacher, 2004). All grafted VU healed without infection or other complications, regrafting or revision in a maximum of 54 days (mean healing time 22 days), with no recurrence during a mean follow-up interval of 19 months. None of these studies distinguished between pain on applying the honey-dressing combination (Dunford and Hanano, 2004), pain between dressing changes and pain on dressing removal.

Results of the two RCTs and two case-controlled series on manuka honey and one non-randomised study of pure natural honey of unspecified origin suggest that there is level A evidence supporting safety of manuka honey, and level C evidence supporting safety of medical grade manuka honey as a primary treatment modality for leg ulcers.

Discussion

The effect of honey on leg ulcers may be more noticeable in those at higher risk of non-healing, simulating a 'kick-start' for recalcitrant leg ulcers. *Figure 10.1* displays the percentage of patients healed in 12 weeks for the three manuka honey studies of VU with different risk levels for non-healing: low (Jull *et al*, 2008), moderate (Gethin, 2008) and high risk, with high risk defined as 12 weeks without healing (Dunford and Hanano, 2004). The healing benefit of manuka honey increased in VU patients less likely to heal during 12 weeks. The clinical implications of this finding are that manuka honey remains effective in the recalcitrant (also called stalled, plateaued or 'stunned' [Ennis and Meneses, 2000]) chronic leg ulcer. The time to consider using manuka honey to restore a leg ulcer to its normal healing path is the moment it becomes clear that the ulcer is not responding to best available practice (Bolton *et al*, 2006), including sustained graduated high compression for venous ulcers. Waiting until a VU deteriorates to become full-thickness before applying evidence-based protocols of care can double its healing time relative to that for a similar area partial-thickness VU (Bolton *et al*, 2004). Proactive wound care professionals will address a recalcitrant leg ulcer as soon as it is recognised. This will improve patient outcomes while minimising resource use.

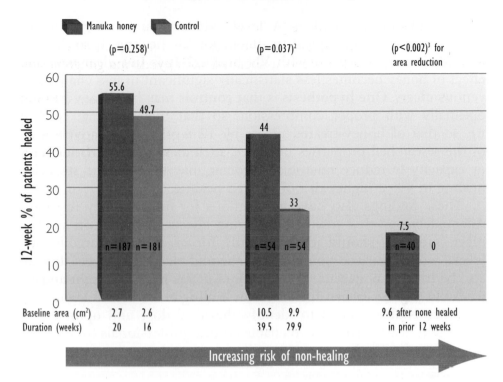

Figure 10.1: Healing effect of honey becomes more consistent with increasing risk of delayed healing. There is a small, non-statistically significant effect of honey in small, short duration venous ulcers with low Margolis risk of delayed healing (1). Honey effect was statistically significant in larger, longer duration venous ulcers (2). Significant 12-week healing occurred in a sample of venous, arterial and mixed venous/arterial ulcers with 100% risk of delayed healing (3), as indicated by failure to respond during the 12 weeks immediately prior to the same treatment regimen without honey. All three studies used honey derived from _Leptospermum scoparium_ (manuka honey).
1. Jull A, Walker N, Parag V, Molan P, Rodgers A (2008) _Br J Surg_ **95**(2): 175–82
2. Gethin G, Cowman S (2008) _J Clin Nurs_ Aug 23 [Epub ahead of print]
3. Dunford CE, Hanano R (2004) _J Wound Care_ **13**(5): 193–7

Trends evident in this chapter generate interesting hypotheses for future research clarifying the effects of honey on wound healing. Further analysis of VU from the two RCTs controlling for variance due to VU duration, size or non-viable tissue on the wound surface may be worthwhile to determine if their combined results corrected for Margolis score provides A level evidence supporting manuka honey as an effective topical treatment for VU healing. If so, how is Margolis score associated with VU healing? It is not clear why the effect of honey becomes less statistically significant in less challenged venous ulcers. One hypothesis is that controls may be already healing optimally with proper compression, so that their healing 'catches up' to that of honey-treated ulcers by 12 weeks. Alternatively, one of the researched properties of honey, such as autolytic debridement or capacity to reduce microbial burdens, may help set the stage for healing in VU at higher risk of delayed healing.

These findings also have implications for future honey research. Adequately powered research clarifying effects of honey on venous ulcer outcomes should ideally stratify for or control Margolis risk levels, wound surface non-viable tissue and ischaemia levels. It may also be fruitful to measure the percent of ulcers healed at eight and 12 weeks to explore earlier differences in healing of lower-risk leg ulcers. Evidence is also needed to identify the ideal dose and optimal top dressing to use over honey to enable clinical professionals to optimise outcomes of using honey as a leg ulcer care modality.

Conclusions

Based on this evidence, one can conclude that level A evidence supports safety and level B evidence supports efficacy of medical grade manuka honey on chronic venous ulcers. Level C evidence supports safety of non-manuka honey as a primary modality for non-venous, non-diabetic, non-malignant leg ulcer treatment. There is currently insufficient evidence to draw a conclusion about the efficacy of manuka honey on non-venous leg ulcers, or of honey from other sources on any type of leg ulcers. While this evidence does begin to clarify the effects of honey on venous ulcers, research is still needed to elucidate the effects on other leg ulcers and wounds, as well as patient, ulcer and care parameters associated with optimal clinical outcomes.

Acknowledgements
The author is especially grateful for the thoughtful review and comments by honey researchers Georgina Gethin and Val Robson and to Rose Cooper and Diane Maydick Youngberg, Clinical Director of Derma Sciences. No commercial support was received in preparing this chapter.

References

Abbade LP, Lastoria S (2005) Venous ulcer: epidemiology, physiopathology, diagnosis and treatment. _Int J Dermatol_ **44**(6): 449–56

Biswal BM, Zakaria A, Ahmad NM (2003) Topical application of honey in the management of radiation mucositis: a preliminary study. _Support Care Cancer_ **11**(4): 242–8

Bolton LL, Corbett L, Bernato DL, Dotson P, Laraus S, Merkle D, _et al_ (2006) Development of a content-validated venous ulcer guideline. _Ostomy/Wound Management_ **52**(11):32–48

Bolton L, McNees P, van Rijswijk L, _et al_ (2004) Wound healing outcomes using standardized care. _JWOCN_ **31**(3): 65–71

Cornwall JV, Dore CJ, Lewis JD (1986) Leg ulcers: epidemiology and aetiology. _Br J Surgery_ **73**: 693–6

Cullum N, Nelson EA, Fletcher AW (2002) The Cochrane library 2001,Compression for venous ulcers (Cochrane Review). In: The Cochrane Library, Issue 3, 2002: Update Software

Dunford CE, Hanano R (2004) Acceptability to patients of a honey dressing for non-healing venous leg ulcers. _J Wound Care_ **13**(5): 193–7

Ennis W, Meneses P (2000) Wound healing at the local level: The stunned wound. _Ostomy/Wound Management_ **46**(suppl 1A): 39S–48S

Gethin G, Cowman S (2008) Manuka honey vs hydrogel — A prospective, open label, multicentre, randomised controlled trial to compare desloughing efficacy and healing outcomes in venous ulcers. _J Clin Nurs_ Aug 23 [Epub ahead of print]

Heit JA, Rooke TW, Silverstein MD, Mohr DN, Lohse CM, Petterson TM, _et al_ (2001) Trends in the incidence of venous stasis syndrome and venous ulcer: a 25-year population-based study. _J Vasc Surgery_ **33**: 1022–7

Jull A, Walker N, Parag V, Molan P, Rodgers A (2008) Honey as adjuvant leg ulcer therapy trial collaborators. Randomized clinical trial of honey-impregnated dressings for venous leg ulcers. _Br J Surg_ **95**(2): 175–82. Comment in: _Evid Based Nurs_ (2008) **11**(3): 87

Leach MJ (2004) Making sense of the venous leg ulcer debate: a literature review. _J Wound Care_ **13**(2): 52–6

Luciana P, Fernandes Abbade MD, Sidnei Lastória MD, Hamilton de Almeida Rollo MD, Hamilton Ometto Stolf MDA (2005) Sociodemographic, clinical study of patients with venous ulcer. _Int J Dermatol_ **44**(12): 989–92

Lyon RT, Veith FJ, Bolton L, Machado F and the Venous Ulcer Study Collaborators (1998) Clincal benchmark for healing of chronic venous ulcers. _Am J Surg_ **176**: 172–5

Margolis D, Berlin J, Strom B (2000) Which venous leg ulcers will heal with limb compression bandages? _Am J Med_ **109**: 15–19

Margolis D, Bilker W, Santanna J, Baumgarten M (2002) Venous leg ulcer: Incidence and prevalence in the elderly. *J Am Acad Dermatol* **46**(3): 381–6

Mashmood AA, Khan TA, Sami AN (2006) Honey compared with 1% silver sulfadiazine cream in the treatment of superficial and partial thickness burns. *J Pakistan Association of Dermatologists* **16**: 14–19

Mekkes JR Loots MAM, Van Der Wall AC, Bos JD (2003) Causes, investigation and treatment of leg ulceration. *Br J Dermatol* **148**: 388–401

Milne C (2008) Use of a honey-impregnated calcium alginate dressing to improve outcomes in pyoderma gangrenosum. Proceedings, Wound Ostomy Continence Nurses Conference, June 21–25, 2008, Orlando

Molan PC (2006) The evidence supporting the use of honey as a wound dressing. *Int J Low Extrem Wounds* **5**(1): 40–54. Erratum in: *Int J Low Extrem Wounds* (2006) **5**(2): 122. Comments in: *Int J Low Extrem Wounds* (2006) **5**(1): 55. *Int J Low Extrem Wounds* (2007) **6**(3): 230

Motallebnejad M, Akram S, Moghadamnia A, Moulana Z, Omidi S (2008) The effect of topical application of pure honey on radiation-induced mucositis: a randomized clinical trial. *J Contemp Dent Pract* **9**(3): 40–7

Oluwatosin OM, Olabanji JK, Oluwatosin OA, Tijani LA, Onyechi HU (2000) A comparison of topical honey and phenytoin in the treatment of chronic leg ulcers. *Afr J Med Med Sci* **29**(1): 31–4

Phillips T, Stanton B, Provan A, Lew R (1994) A study of the impact of leg ulcers on quality of life: Financial, social and psychological implications. *J Am Acad Dermatol* **31**: 49–53

Registered Nurses Association of Ontario (2005) *Risk assessment and prevention of pressure ulcers*. RNAO, Toronto

Romanelli M (1997) Objective measurement of venous ulcer debridement and granulation with a skin color reflectance analyzer. *Wounds* **9**(4): 122–6

Schumacher HH (2004) Use of medical honey in patients with chronic venous leg ulcers after split-skin grafting. *J Wound Care* **13**(10): 451–2

Wipke-Tevis DD, Sae-Sia W (2005) Management of vascular leg ulcers. *Adv Skin Wound Care* **18**: 437–45

Wound, Ostomy, and Continence Nurses Society (WOCN) (2003) *Guideline for prevention and management of pressure ulcers*. Wound, Ostomy, and Continence Nurses Society (WOCN), Glenview (IL). Available online at: www.guideline.gov (last accessed 1 July, 2008)

Chapter 11

Honey in Paediatric Care and Oncology

Arne Simon, Gisela Blaser and Kai Santos

Six years ago a twelve-year-old patient was submitted to our unit (the Children's Hospital Medical Centre, University of Bonn, Germany). Doctors at another hospital had partially removed an intra-abdominal lymphoma, leaving an open drainage site on the child's abdominal wall. On admission, the wound was infected with methicillin-resistant *Staphylococcus aureus* (MRSA). To avoid nosocomial spread, the patient was immediately kept under contact isolation, a difficult situation for the child to understand and significant additional costs for the hospital. Although the patient was scheduled to receive chemotherapy, treatment could not start until the infection had cleared. The wound was treated with a local antiseptic (octenidine) for twelve days. However, as there was no improvement, our wound care specialist decided to use an Australian medical honey product (Medihoney™), containing *Leptospermum* honey, which has excellent *in vitro* activity against MRSA (Cooper *et al*, 1999; Cooper *et al*, 2002; Lusby *et al*, 2005, Blaser *et al*, 2007). Two days later, the wound was free of bacteria and the chemotherapy against the underlying illness could be started.

In our paediatric oncology department at the Children's Hospital Medical Centre, most patients suffer from a suppressed immune system due to their underlying illness (i.e. leukaemia) (Lehrnbecher *et al*, 1997) and the chemotherapy that they undergo. This frequently results in wound-healing problems (Simon *et al*, 2006; Gaur *et al*, 2005) leaving the patient susceptible to wound infections. Unfortunately, in these patients local infections spread easily and can cause secondary, potentially life-threatening bloodstream infections (Gaur *et al*, 2004). This chapter will outline the reasons why the topical use of medical honey has become integrated into our wound treatment strategies.

Antiseptic properties of medical honey

In our unit, a common treatment for critically colonised or infected wounds before the implementation of medical honey had been povidone iodine. This topical agent has the advantage of antiseptic properties and it is well suited for skin disinfection prior to invasive procedures. However, the antiseptic activity of iodine products is hampered by interactions with the protein content of wound exudate and severe adverse effects of systemic absorption of iodine on thyroid function (Shetty and Duthie, 1990; Meurisse *et al*, 2000). This limitation must be considered in infants and toddlers, as well as in adult patients with latent hyperthyroidism. In contrast, medical honey does not have the problem of systemic absorption and thus it can even be utilised in patients with diabetes mellitus without adverse effects on blood glucose levels (Eddy and Gideonsen, 2005; Yaghoobi *et al*, 2008).

Normally an ideal wound antiseptic would be expected to meet the following criteria (Kramer *et al*, 2004):

- fast onset of bactericidal action and a remnant, broad spectrum effect against bacteria and fungi, even under the unfavourable conditions of exudating, colonised or infected wounds
- enhancement and acceleration of the physiologic process of wound healing (debridement, granulation), even if applied for prolonged periods
- no adverse local or systemic effects (allergy, toxicity related to absorption).

Medical honey (all our experiences refer to Medihoney™) meets all of the above criteria except 'a fast onset of activity', as it does not seem to produce the desired reduction of bacteria and fungi (more than five log units in 1–10 minutes) to allow it to be qualified as an antiseptic. Nevertheless, we have used it successfully to eradicate MRSA from infected wounds (Blaser *et al*, 2007), and we have used it prophylactically at catheter entry sites.

Medihoney™ treatment in the setting of allogenic stem cell transplantation

An adult patient with acute myeloic leukaemia in relapse had a wound infection after thoracic surgery for invasive *Aspergillus* infection of

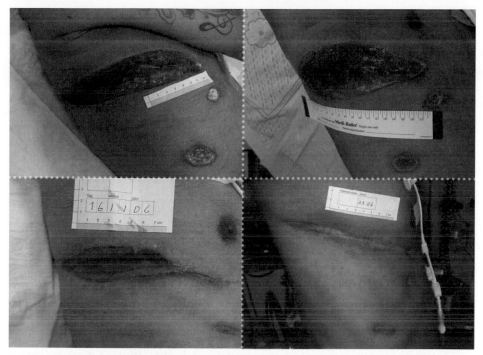

Figure 11.1: A 26 year old patient with acute mycloic leukaemia (relapse); post-surgical wound infection with methicillin-resistant *Staphylococcus epidermidis* after thoracotomy (resection of an aspergilloma of the right upper right lobe). Wound care included Medihoney™ plus calcium-alginate dressing for seven weeks (during allogeneic stem cell tx)

the lung, but was allocated to allogenic bone marrow transplantation. Using Medihoney™ the wound infection was eliminated. The patient continued to receive Medihoney™ applications during and after the transplant (*Figure 11.1*), leading to successful healing without further local or systemic complications.

Medihoney™ for the protection of catheter entry sites

The clinical usefulness of haemodialysis catheters is limited by the risk of infection causing increased morbidity and mortality. Topical antiseptic agents, such as mupirocin, are effective at reducing this risk but have been reported to select for antibiotic-resistant strains (Cookson, 1998). Honey has not yet been reported to select for resistant strains (Blair and Carter, 2005).

Johnson *et al* (2005) performed a randomised, controlled trial comparing the effect of thrice-weekly exit-site application of Medihoney™ versus mupirocin on infection rates in patients who were receiving haemodialysis via tunnelled, cuffed central venous catheters. A total of 101 patients were enrolled. The incidences of catheter-associated bacteraemia in honey-treated ($n=51$) and mupirocin-treated ($n=50$) patients were comparable (0.97 versus 0.85 episodes per 1000 catheter-days, respectively; NS). No exit-site infections occurred. During the study period, 2% of staphylococcal isolates within the hospital were mupirocin resistant. Thrice-weekly application of standardised antibacterial honey to haemodialysis catheter exit sites was safe, cheap and effective, and resulted in a comparable rate of catheter-associated infection to that obtained with mupirocin (although the study was not adequately powered to assess therapeutic equivalence).

The effectiveness of honey against antibiotic-resistant micro-organisms and its low likelihood of selecting for further resistant strains suggest that this agent may represent a satisfactory alternative means of local (entry site) prophylaxis in patients with central venous catheters. In our paediatric oncology unit, all entry sites of tunnelled central venous catheters, which show any sign of inflammation or dehiscence, are routinely covered with Medihoney™. Another important indication for the use of medical honey is the secondary healing of deep wound pockets, which result from the removal of an infected port catheter (central venous access device with a subcutaneously implanted reservoir) (*Figure 11.2*).

Additional benefits of medical honey to wound care

The debriding action of honey has been noted by many (Molan, 2002), this would be expected to help in removing slough which is a rich source of the bacteria that stimulate an inflammatory response (Molan, 2002). With hospitals facing increasing problems of bacterial resistance, it is important to note that the use of medical honey has been observed neither to foster bacterial resistance (Blair and Carter, 2005), nor to have any toxic effects after prolonged periods of application (Molan, 2002; Johnson *et al*, 2005).

Medical honey eases the procedure of dressing changes, in particular in paediatric patients, who are unable to accept any pain related to this procedure (Dunford *et al*, 2000). With medical honey, systemic analgosedation (an elaborate and sometimes risky procedure)

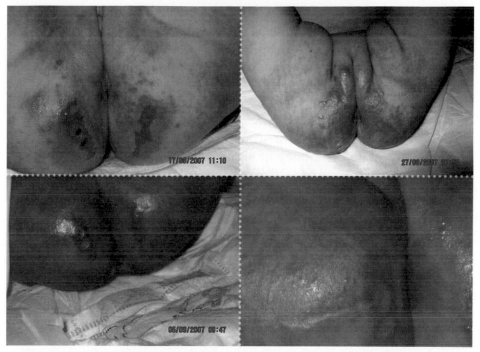

Figure 11.2: An eight-month-old female infant with acute myeloic leukaemia and sepsis (*Pseudomonas aeruginosa*) during granulocytopenia. Wound care included cleaning with sterile Ringer-solution, 10 x 10 cm calcium-alginate dressing plus Medihoney™ (four weeks)

is no longer necessary for dressing changes in most instances. Another important benefit is that medical honey successfully manages the problem of malodour from chronic colonised wounds, which can cause patients severe discomfort and social isolation (Molan, 1999).

Honey for mucositis and oral care

Ingestion of honey seems to offer potential in treating mucositosis. Many cancer patients suffer from mucositis, a side-effect of chemotherapy that attacks the entire gastrointestinal tract from the mouth to the anus (Blijlevens, 2007). The cancer treatment breaks down the epithelial cells lining the tract, leaving patients prone to ulcerations and infections. These important and beneficial cells replicate and divide rapidly, which is why in a typical healthy individual wounds in the mouth heal quickly. Chemotherapy does not distinguish between healthy and malignant cells, attacking all that reproduce rapidly, including these epithelial cells.

Twenty to forty percent of all cancer patients receiving intensive chemotherapy suffer from mucositis, the number climbs to 80% when chemotherapy and radiation are combined, and staggers even higher in patients receiving treatment for cancer in the head and neck area.

Open sores in cancer patients suffering from mucositis leave them susceptible to infection. In a study conducted in 2003, Biswal *et al* investigated the use of honey in 40 adult patients with head and neck cancer. Patients consumed 20 ml (1 1/3 teaspoon) of pure honey 15 minutes before, 15 minutes after and six hours post-treatment. There was significant reduction in the symptomatic grade 3/4 mucositis (which describes the necessity for morphine infusion and parenteral nutrition) among honey-treated patients compared with controls, i.e. 20% versus 75% ($p < 0.001$). The compliance of the honey-treated group of patients was better than controls. Fifty-five percent of patients treated with topical honey showed no change or a positive gain in body weight compared to only 25% in the control arm ($p = 0.05$).

Another recently published study investigated the use of honey as topical prophylaxis against radio-chemotherapy-induced mucositis in head and neck cancer (Rashad *et al*, 2008). The study was performed in Assiut University Hospital, Egypt, between January 2005 and July 2006. Forty patients diagnosed with head and neck cancer were entered into the trial. Enrolled patients were randomised to the treatment group, receiving concomitant chemotherapy and radiotherapy (with a significant area of directly visible oral and/or oropharyngeal mucosa included in the radiation fields), plus prior topical application of pure natural honey, or the control group, receiving concomitant chemotherapy and radiotherapy without honey. Patients were evaluated clinically every week to assess development of radiation mucositis. Aerobic cultures and *Candida* colonisation assessments were undertaken via oral and oropharyngeal swabs, prior to and at the completion of irradiation, and when infection was evident. In the treatment group, no patients developed WHO IV mucositis (intravenous morphine, parenteral nutrition) and only three patients (15%) developed WHO III mucositis. In the control group, 13 patients (65%) developed WHO III or IV mucositis ($p < 0.05$). *Candida* colonisation was found in 15% of the treatment group and 60% of the control group, either during or after radiotherapy ($p = 0.003$). Positive cultures for aerobic pathogenic bacteria were observed in 15% of the treatment group and 65% of the control group, during or after radiotherapy ($p = 0.007$).

According to a review, honey has potential for the treatment of periodontal disease, mouth ulcers and other problems of oral health (Molan, 2001), and a trial has demonstrated a statistically significant difference between chewing gelled honey and chewing chewing-gum in decreasing the number of bleeding sites on gums with gingivitis (English *et al*, 2004).

Compliance issues with medical honey

Dunford and Hanan (2004) undertook a four-centre feasibility study to determine whether Medihoney™ is an acceptable treatment for patients with leg ulcers in terms of pain relief, odour control and overall patient satisfaction. Forty patients whose leg ulcers had not responded to 12 weeks of compression therapy were recruited. Medihoney dressings were applied on their ulcers for the 12-week study period. All other aspects of their care, including the use of compression bandaging, remained unchanged. Overall, ulcer pain and size decreased significantly and malodorous wounds were deodorised promptly.

These results revealed a high patient acceptance for this treatment. The same first author reported the care of an adolescent with multiple wounds, infected with resistant bacterial pathogens after meningococcal sepsis and limb amputation (Dunford *et al*, 2000). Before the use of medical honey, each dressing change had to be performed under general anaesthesia to alleviate pain and anxiety. Shortly after the introduction of medical honey dressings, the wounds improved and dressing changes could be performed without any analgesic medication. We have had similar experiences with children in our clinic. If the Medihoney™ dressing is completely moistened with sterile Ringer's solution, it can easily and painlessly be removed without any attachment to the wound. In our unit and our wound care ambulance, parents or relatives are educated in the aseptic procedure of the dressing change and are able to perform it at home.

Adverse effects with honey

There are two important adverse events related to the use of medical honey. About 5% of the authors' patients experience stinging pain after the application honey. This problem may be avoided by conditioning the wound surface with a sterile anaesthetic cream. Unfortunately, local anaesthetics cause vasoconstriction. Thus, this method may result in an objectionable reduction of local perfusion. In some patients who experienced such pain, treatment with medical honey had to be stopped or postponed until the acute inflammatory process had been controlled by other treatment approaches, for example, irrigation and gel containing polyhexanide (Horrocks, 2006).

Two of more than 150 patients from our patient population showed reproducible local atopic reactions to Medihoney™. Both children had an underlying atopic disposition. We are not aware of any severe systemic atopic reactions related to the use of medical honey from either our experience or from the published literature.

Practical considerations

Medical honey dressings should keep the honey in contact with the wound for at least 12 hours, preferably 24 hours. Some patients apply the wound dressing overnight, so as not to restrict their mobility during the day. If the dressing is inappropriate, the honey may be washed out of the wound by exudate. This may be a practical problem and a challenge in some wounds, as was found in a post-surgical wound (deep abscess of the pilonidal sinus directly above the natal cleft) in one of our patients, who was treated for a Ewing sarcoma of the pelvis (*Figure 11.3*).

The clinical benefits of medical honey, including antibacterial protection, wound cleaning and pH modulation may, as a result, be reduced. From our experience (Simon *et al*, 2006) and the experience of others (White *et al*, 2005), the best way to keep the honey in the wound is to soak medical honey into a moistened (sterile NaCl 0.9%) calcium-alginate or hydrofiber dressing, which forms a gel with the honey as it absorbs the exudate.

In case of an infected wound, a hospital grade, licensed antiseptic (e.g. octenidine) is applied to infected wounds in addition to Medihoney™ on the first two days of treatment. Severely immunocompromised patients with neutropenia (neutrophil count $< 0.5 \times 09/l$ or leukocyte counts $< 1 \times 109/l$ and no differential count available) have to be treated concomitantly with systemic antibiotics in case of fever or any sign of local soft tissue infection.

For safety reasons, wound care with medical honey should always be supervised by a physician or a wound care specialist in patients with chronic, complicated wounds or with significant comorbidities. The 'honey approach' to wound care must be part of a comprehensive wound care concept. Any comorbidity which contributes to the problems in wound healing should be diagnosed and treated thoroughly (e.g. bypass surgery in patients with reduced arterial perfusion, compression bandages in patients with chronic venous ulcers, control of blood glucose levels in patients with diabetic food syndrome) (Gethin and Cowman, 2005). The frequency of dressing changes depends on the amount of exudate. In the early stages, fresh surgical wounds infected with pathogenic bacteria may need twice-daily dressing changes.

In more persistent wound care situations, Medihoney™ dressings have been left in place for up to seven days (Gethin and Cowman, 2005; Gethin, 2004) and a mean initial wound size for all wounds of $5.62 \, \text{cm}^2$ was obtained. At the end of a four-week treatment period, the mean size was $2.25 \, \text{cm}^2$. Odour was eliminated and pain reduced. The

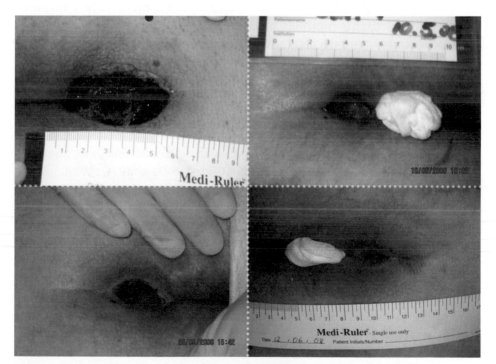

Figure 11.3: A 20-year-old patient with Ewing sarcoma of the pelvis. Abscess (sinus pinoidalis) developed during severe chemotherapy-induced granulcytopenia and thrombocytopenia. Wound care included Medihoney™ plus Aquacel® (two months)

conclusions drawn were that the use of manuka honey was associated with a positive wound-healing outcome in these eight cases. Arterial wounds showed minimal improvement only (Gethin *et al*, 2005). Prospective studies confirming the efficacy of extended dressing change intervals are not yet available.

Some of the parents and, indeed, doctors in our unit have at first been sceptical about the benefits of medical honey in wound care. Some colleagues questioned the scientific evidence of this approach. However, the scientific evidence for using conventional wound care products in paediatric oncology patients is non-existent, since no prospective randomised studies have been performed in this particular population and no research has been done on the long-term effects of modern conventional treatments, such as silver dressings (Trop *et al*, 2006). Taken together, the scientific evidence for using medical honey in wound care is impressive (Molan, 2006) and, thus, medical honey should not be 'the last resort' for recalcitrant wound care situations (Simon *et al*, 2008).

It is important that the wound care team objectively evaluates the benefit of using medical honey each dressing change. In cases where wounds show no movement, signs of local intolerance (severe pain after administration), or is even getting worse while being treated with medical honey, diagnostic swabs for microbiologic investigation should be collected and the treatment regimen changed, for example, to flush solutions and dressings containing polyhexanide as an antiseptic.

Cost issues

In settings where wound treatment is not covered by health insurance, the cost of medical honey treatment, such as Medihoney™, cannot be afforded by most patients. However, in many countries, medical honey products can now be prescribed, as with other professional wound dressings.

Prospective studies investigating the overall cost of treatment with medical honey compared with conventional wound care approaches are awaited (Simon *et al*, 2008). In chronic recalcitrant wounds, the most cost-effective treatment is, obviously, the one which eventually results in wound healing. Many of the wound care patients we have treated with medical honey had previously received specialist attention for recalcitrant wounds for months or even for years. When treatment with honey was started, the wound status changed to healing from non-healing in the majority of cases. Similar findings have been reported by others (Cooper *et al*, 2001; Molan, 2002; Simon *et al*, 2006; Blaser *et al*, 2007).

Clostridium spores

In deep wound cavities the possibility exists of an anaerobic environment, where *Clostridium botulinum* spores could proliferate and produce botulinum toxin. Negative effects such as paralysis and cardiac arrhythmia have been described related to systemic effects of the toxin. To eliminate botulism spores with heat, honey would need to be heated to 120°C (248°F) for 10 minutes, which would result in adverse changes to some of the beneficial properties of honey.

Since spores have occasionally been found in honey, all modern licensed wound care products containing honey are gamma-irradiated to inactivate spores, such as those from *Clostridium* sp. Irradiation does not have a detrimental impact on the antibacterial activity of honey (Molan and Allen, 1996).

Due to our experience of the safety of Medihoney™ with infants, we are using this product for wound care in premature neonates. One such patient had a recalcitrant wound after surgical intervention for myelomeningocele. The wound stagnated and during intensive care treatment it became colonised with multi-resistant *Klebsiella oxytoca*. Before treatment with Medihoney™ was initiated, the child had received numerous intravenous antibiotics and many other conventional wound care treatments to clear the wound, spending the first three months of its life in the hospital. Medihoney™ dressings cleared the wound of the pathogen and allowed the patient to be discharged after three weeks. The wound healed completely without further surgical intervention (*Figure 11.4*).

WoundViewer© POMS

We recently developed a database (WoundViewer©, Children's Hospital, University of Bonn, Germany) for the standardised collection of datasets concerning the clinical use of Medihoney™ products in wound care to allow the collection of clinical evidence and to support the design of prospective comparative studies in the

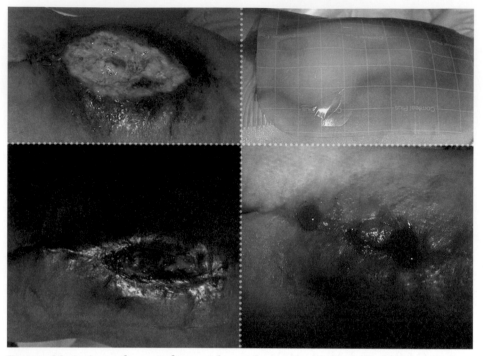

Figure 11.4: A newborn infant with myelomeningocele and recalcitrant postsurgical wound infection (three months) with multi-resistant *Klebsiella oxytoca*. Closure of the wound was achieved with Medihoney™ plus a hydrocolloid and outpatient treatment started after three weeks

near future. In 2009, the results of a multicentre post-marketing surveillance study using this software in 15 wound care centres in Germany will be available.

Conclusion

In conclusion, the routine use of medical honey (Medihoney™) in a broad clinical spectrum of acute and chronic wounds has improved our efforts to hasten wound healing and protect the highly immunocompromised patients from secondary infections.

The dressing changes are easy to perform and we noticed a reduction in the need for analgosediation related to this procedure. From our perspective, the use of medical honey should be included as one standard alternative to other wound care approaches.

Acknowledgement

We would like to dedicate this chapter with our thanks to the head of our paediatric oncology department, Professor Dr Udo Bode, for all his help over the past ten years.

References

Biswal BM, Zakaria A, Ahmad NM (2003) Topical application of honey in the management of radiation mucositis: a preliminary study. *Support Care Cancer* 11(4): 242–8

Blair S, Carter D (2005) The potential for honey in the management of wound and infection. *J Aus Infect Control* 10(1): 24–31

Blijlevens NM (2007) Cytotoxic treatment-induced gastrointestinal symptoms. *Curr Opin Support Palliat Care* 1(1): 16–22

Blaser G, Santos K, Bode U, Vetter H, Simon A (2007) Treatment of MRSA colonized or infected wounds with Medihoney™ antibacterial honey products. *J Wound Care* 16(8):325–8

Canter PH, Coon JT, Ernst E (2006) Cost-effectiveness of complementary therapies in the United Kingdom — a systematic review. *Evid Based Complement Alternat Med* 3(4): 425–32

Cookson BD (1998) The emergence of mupirocin resistance: a challenge to infection control and antibiotic prescribing practice. *J Antimicrob Chemother* 41(1): 11–18

Cooper RA, Molan PC, Harding KG (1999) Antibacterial activity of honey against strains of *Staphylococcus aureus* from infected wounds. *J R Soc Med* 92(6): 283–5

Cooper RA, Molan PC, Krishnamoorthy L, Harding KG (2001) Manuka honey used to heal a recalcitrant surgical wound. *Eur J Clin Microbiol Infect Dis* 20(10): 758–9

Cooper RA, Molan PC, Harding KG (2002) The sensitivity to honey of Gram-positive cocci of clinical significance isolated from wounds. *J Appl Microbiol* 93(5):857–63

Dunford C, Cooper R, Molan P (2000) Using honey as a dressing for infected skin lesions. *Nurs Times* 96(14 Suppl): 7–9

Dunford CE, Hanano R (2004) Acceptability to patients of a honey dressing for non-healing venous leg ulcers. J Wound Care 13(5): 193–7

Eddy JJ, Gideonsen MD (2005) Topical honey for diabetic foot ulcers. *J Fam Pract* 54(6): 533–5

English H, Pack A, Molan P (2004) The effects of manuka honey on plaque and gingivitis: a pilot study. *J Int Acad Periodontol* 6(2): 63–7

Gaur AH, Flynn PM, Shenep JL (2004) Optimum management of pediatric patients with fever and neutropenia. *Indian J Pediatr* 71(9): 825–35

Gaur AH, Liu T, Knapp KM, Daw NC, Rao BN, Neel MD, *et al* (2005) Infections in children and young adults with bone malignancies undergoing limb-sparing surgery. *Cancer* 104(3): 602–10

Gethin G (2004) Is there enough clinical evidence to use honey to manage wounds? *J Wound Care* 13(7): 275–8

Gethin G, Cowman S (2005) Case series of use of Manuka honey in leg ulceration. *Int Wound J* 2(1): 10–5

Horrocks A (2006) Prontosan wound irrigation and gel: management of chronic wounds. *Br J Nurs* 15(22): 1222, 1224–8

Johnson DW, van Eps C, Mudge DW, Wiggins KJ, Armstrong K, Hawley CM, *et al* (2005) Randomized, controlled trial of topical exit-site application of honey (Medihoney) versus mupirocin for the prevention of catheter-associated infections in hemodialysis patients. *J Am Soc Nephrol* 16(5): 1456–62

Kramer A, Daeschlein G, Kammerlander G, Abdriessen A, Aspöck C, Bergemann R, *et al* (2004) Consensus recommendation for the choice of antiseptic agents in wound care (Article in German). *Hygiene und Medizin* 29(5): 147–57

Lehrnbecher T, Foster C, Vazquez N, Mackall CL, Chanock SJ (1997) Therapy-induced alterations in host defense in children receiving therapy for cancer. *J Pediatr Hematol Oncol* 19(5): 399–417

Lusby PE, Coombes AL, Wilkinson JM (2005) Bactericidal activity of different honeys against pathogenic bacteria. *Arch Med Res* 36(5): 464–7

Meurisse M, Gollogly I, Degauque C, *et al* (2000) Iatrogenic thyrotoxicosis: causal circumstances, pathophysiology, and principles of treatment — review of the literature. *World J Surg* 24(11): 1377–85

Molan PC (1999) The role of honey in the management of wounds. *J Wound Care* 8(8): 415–8

Molan PC (2001) The potential of honey to promote oral wellness. *Gen Dent* 49(6): 584–9

Molan PC (2002) Re-introducing honey in the management of wounds and ulcers — theory and practice. *Ostomy Wound Manage* 48(11): 28–40

Molan PC (2006) The evidence supporting the use of honey as a wound dressing. *Int J Low Extrem Wounds* 5(1): 40–54

Molan PC, Allen KL (1996) The effect of gamma-irradiation on the antibacterial activity of honey. *J Pharm Pharmacol* 48(11): 1206–9

Rashad UM, Al-Gezawy SM, El-Gezawy E, Azzaz AN (2008) Honey as topical prophylaxis against radio chemotherapy-induced mucositis in head and neck cancer. *J Laryngol Otol* May 19: 1–6. [Epub ahead of print]

Shetty KR, Duthie EH (1990) Thyrotoxicosis induced by topical iodine application. *Arch Intern Med* 150(11): 2400–1

Simon A, Sofka K, Wiszniewsky G, Blaser G, Bode U, Fleischhack G (2006) Wound care with antibacterial honey (Medihoney) in pediatric hematology-oncology.

Support Care Cancer **14**(1): 91–7

Simon A, Traynor K, Santos K, Blaser G, Bode U, Molan PC (2008) Medical Honey for wound care — still the 'latest resort'? *Evid Based Complement Alternat Med* (eCAM) 2008; 5(eCAM advance access published January 7, 2008)

Trop M, Novak M, Rodl S, Hellbom B, Kroell W, Goessler W (2006) Silver-coated dressing acticoat caused raised liver enzymes and argyria-like symptoms in burn patient. *J Trauma* **60**(3): 648–52

White R, Cooper R, Molan PC, eds (2005) *Honey: a modern wound management product*. Wounds UK, Aberdeen, UK

Yaghoobi N, Al-Waili N, Ghayour-Mobarhan M, *et al* (2008) Natural honey and cardiovascular risk factors: effects on blood glucose, cholesterol, triacylglycerol, CRP and body weight. *Scientific World* **8**: 463–9

Chapter 12

Honey and Radiotherapy Damaged Tissue

Val Robson

Radiotherapy is a major modality in the treatment of cancer. More than 50% of all cancer patients receive some form of radiotherapy for tumour control pre- or post-operatively (Bentzen and Overgaard, 1994; Holmes, 1988; Mendelsohn *et al*, 2002). Even though radiotherapy is targeted at a particular location and depth, tissues overlying the site can also be affected and may react to the treatment, this happens in about 95% of patients (De Conno *et al*, 1991; Porock and Kristjanson, 1999).

Over the past 30 years the International Agency for Research on Cancer (IARC) has prepared estimates of the global cancer burden. This estimate included 10.9 million new cases of cancer globally for 2002 (Parkin *et al*, 2005). The most recent incidence and mortality data on which these estimates have been based are from the period between 1993 and 2001.It is estimated in England and Wales that one in three people will develop cancer during their lifetime. In 2005, 239,000 new cases of malignant cancer (excluding non-melanoma skin cancer) were registered (National Statistics, www.statistics.gov. uk). In Scotland 36,509 new cases were registered in 2005 (NHS Scotland, National Services Scotland, www.isdscotland.org). Each year the American Cancer Society (ACS) estimates the number of new cancer cases expected in the United States (USA) and for 2007, based on incidence data through to 2003 and mortality data through to 2004, a projected total of 1,444,920 new cases were anticipated (Jemel *et al*, 2007).

Survival rate for cancer was estimated globally in 2002 as 24.6 million alive with cancer within three years of diagnosis (Parkin *et al*, 2005). Cancer survival in England and Wales for 1996–1999 (for all cancers combined) confirm that the five-year relative survival rate has now reached 50% (Office for National Statistics, 2003). In

Scotland, the five-year relative survival, taking all cancers combined, for the period 2000–2004 is 42% for males and 51% for females (NHS Scotland, National Services Scotland). From the National Cancer Institute, USA, Surveillance Epidemiology and End Results (SEER) data for 1996–2004 in the USA, 65.3% of people were five-year survivors (Surveillance Epidemiology and End Results, www.seer. cancer.gov). Although geographical, race, age and sex variations exist, it is a fair estimate that half the long-term survivors will have had radiotherapy as a primary treatment or in combination with surgery and/or chemotherapy (Bentzen and Overgaard, 1994). Delaney _et al_ (2005) pointed out that 52% of cancer patients are expected to receive radiotherapy and estimated that for 40% of those patients surviving at least five years, radiotherapy had contributed either alone, or in combination with other treatments and surgery, to their survival Delaney _et al_, 2005).

Radiation damage

Radiation tissue damage or injury refers to the morphological and functional changes that occur in non-cancerous tissue as a direct result of ionising radiation (Mendelsohn _et al_, 2002). Radiotherapy induces the formation of free radicals and peroxides which effect adverse changes in DNA, proteins and cellular membranes. Although cells have scavenging mechanisms to remove these dangerous free radicals, repeated bouts of radiation overwhelm them. DNA may be affected by breaks in either single or double strands, and cross-linking between strands may develop. Repair enzymes normally operate to remove these changes. If the damage is extensive, repair may not be successfully completed and cells die by apoptosis. If repair is effected, normal cell function is retrieved, but incomplete restoration leads to permanent changes (or mutations) that give rise to dysfunctional cells. The acute side-effects are greatest in cells that are actively dividing such as skin, bone marrow and gastrointestinal mucosa (Porock and Kristjanson, 1999). Severity of the adverse effects of radiation is dependent upon the radiosensitivity of the body sites being treated, the total dose and the rate of accumulation of cellular defects (Porock, 2002; Denham and Hauer-Jensen, 2002; Stone _et al_, 2003).

There are parts of skin that have an elevated risk of damage, such as where two skin surfaces are in contact (e.g. breast, perineum), or areas where the epidermis is thin and smooth (e.g. axillae, face, perineum), or sites where the skin integrity has already been damaged (e.g. from surgery, burns or lesions) (McQuestion, 2006). Comorbidities such as diabetes, renal failure, hypertension, age, compromised nutritional status, smoking, drug therapy, chemotherapy and skin colour may also affect the tissue reaction to radiotherapy. Furthermore, it is suggested that some patients may have a genetic susceptibility to the developing radiation injury. Patients with ataxia telangiectasia develop severe reactions because of the defect in the repair of DNA after exposure to radiotherapy (Porock, 2002; Stone *et al*, 2003; McQuestion, 2006).

Response to radiotherapy

The normal response to traumatic injury involves a complex cascade of events involving:

- haemostasis (immediate)
- inflammation (day 0–4)
- granulation tissue formation (day 3–3 weeks)
- matrix deposition and remodelling (week 3–2 years)
  (Denham and Hauer-Jensen, 2002; Dormand *et al*, 2005).

Many responses/effects following radiotherapy damage are similar to those following traumatic injury. However, the accumulating and repetitive damage during the course of treatment affects the 'normal' tissue that is within the radiation field. Thus, 'normal' tissue that was irradiated at the start of treatment is qualitatively very different to that same tissue when it is irradiated later (Denham and Hauer-Jensen, 2002).

Radiation injury is commonly classified as acute, late effects and consequential late effects according to the time before appearance of symptoms.

Acute effects

Radiotherapy leads to apoptotic cell death in malignant and healthy cells within the radiation field, as well as multiple cellular effects in surviving cells (Stone *et al*, 2003; Dormand *et al*, 2005; Maddocks-Jennings *et al*, 2005). The physical trauma results in the activation of an acute inflammatory response (Dormand *et al*, 2005), although the changes that occur in the skin can start within hours of treatment, they may last for several months or even be permanent (Maddocks-Jennings *et al*, 2005). During the first two weeks of treatment the patient may experience soreness, erythema and/or burning, and the area may be sensitive and feel tight. If the total radiation dose to the skin does not exceed approximately 30 Gy (Gy, the measure of radiation dose), the erythema phase is followed during the fourth or fifth week by a dry desquamation phase, characterised by pruritus, scaling, and an increase in melanin pigmentation in the basal layer. Within two months, inflammatory exudate and oedema subside, leaving an area of pigmentation. If the total radiation dose to the skin is 40 Gy or greater, the erythema phase is followed by a 'moist' desquamation phase. This stage usually begins in the fourth week and is often accompanied by considerable discomfort. Bullous formation occurs, the roofs of the bullae are shed and the entire epidermis may be lost in portions of the irradiated area. Oedema and fibrinous exudate persist. In the absence of infection, re-epithelialisation usually begins within 10 days. Ulcers may appear at any time from approximately two weeks after radiation exposure. Ulcers formed in the early stage are a result of direct necrosis of the epidermis, these ulcers usually heal but tend to recur (Mendelsohn *et al*, 2002; Dormand *et al*, 2005; Maddocks-Jennings *et al*, 2005; McQuestion, 2006).

Late effects

Late effects develop months or years after treatment including necrosis, atrophy, fibrosis, vascular damage and carcinogenesis. Late effects tend to develop in tissues with a slow turnover of cells, such as subcutaneous tissue, fatty tissue, muscle, brain, kidney and liver (Stone *et al*, 2003). Non-healing ulcers may develop at any time following radiotherapy and up to decades afterwards (Dormand *et al*, 2005). A report has already been published of a case where the use of honey on a chronic wound that had developed on tissue damaged by radiotherapy 30 years earlier promoted successful healing (Robson *et al*, 2005).

Consequential late effects

In some patients acute reactions fail to heal completely. Consequential late effects are increasingly being observed because of the introduction of new aggressive treatment regimes with combined modalities, such as radiotherapy and chemotherapy (Stone *et al*, 2003).

Treatment options for radiation tissue damage

Currently, there is little objective evidence to support the use of any interventions or products that are currently available for the care and treatment of radiotherapy skin reactions. A survey that was completed in 1992 with information collected from 31 radiotherapy centres, hospices, and community and specialist nurses in the United Kingdom found that of the 112 individuals who responded, 69.6% had used creams or ointments on radiotherapy damaged skin. From those practitioners, a total of 40 different topical products were identified. Comparatively fewer responses were received in relation to the use of dressings for the management of radiation damaged skin. Only 17 dressings were identified and when asked which dressings were thought to be unsuitable for this kind of wound care, 17 products were specified. Some of the dressings promoted by some respondents were considered unsuitable by others. The author of the survey inferred that the observations suggested either dissatisfaction with the dressings that were available or a failure to appreciate the advantages of newer dressings (Thomas, 1992).

At present, irradiated wounds are cared for in a similar manner to other chronic wounds because their exact microenvironment has not yet been fully characterised (Hom *et al*, 1999). Accurate holistic assessment of the wound is advised. Adequate debridement followed by a dressing that promotes granulation tissue formation has been recommended; adhesive dressings are avoided to prevent epithelial injury (Hom *et al*, 1999). A recently published review of the literature recommends topical antimicrobial therapy with antiseptics to prevent infection in radiotherapy ulcers (Olascoaga *et al*, 2008).

There are numerous small studies making various recommendations such as hydrocolloid dressings (Margolin *et al*, 1990; Mak *et al*, 2000), topical negative pressure (TNP) (Schimp *et al*, 2004), hyperbaric oxygen (Borg *et al*, 2001), and Mepilex® Lite soft silicone dressing (Mölnlycke Health Care) (MacBride *et al*, 2008). A study in the Netherlands on 24 patients who suffered skin reactions from radiotherapy were randomised into two groups. The control group received a paraffin gauze dressing and the study group had honey-impregnated gauze applied. Although no statistical significance was found, the authors concluded that the honey group displayed a trend towards faster healing of skin reactions and had greater patient satisfaction (Moolenaar et al, 2006).

Three clinical studies have advocated the use of honey in the management of radiation mucositis in patients with head and neck cancer receiving radiation to the oropharyngeal mucosal area. In one study, 40 patients were divided into two equal groups. The control group received radiotherapy alone and the study group received radiotherapy plus topical honey. A significant reduction in the symptomatic grade 3/4 mucositis was seen in honey-treated patients compared to the control group (Biswal et al, 2003). In a similar study of 40 patients, significantly reduced mucositis, as assessed by the Oral Mucositis Assessment Scale (OMAS), in the honey-treated patients was reported. Compared with a normal saline rinse, honey before and after radiotherapy was found to give statistically significant reduction in OMAS throughout a six-week treatment period (Motallebnejad et al, 2008). In a third study on head and neck cancer patients, 40 patients were randomised to receive honey or no-treatment as a prophylactic measure. Oral and pharyngeal mucositis were assessed, and, oropharyngeal swabs were cultured for aerobic bacteria and _Candida_ spp. In the honey-treated group, fewer patients developed mucositis ($p < 0.05$) and fewer positive cultures for either _Candida_ spp. ($p = 0.003$) or aerobes ($p = 0.007$) were reported, compared to the untreated group (Rashad et al, 2008).

Honey seems to offer potential in the treatment of radiation damaged tissue in several ways. It is a broad spectrum antimicrobial agent that has the potential not only to prevent infection, but also to eradicate bacteria from wounds (Cooper, 2008). Since infection is a possible complication in such tissue (Hom et al, 1999), the antimicrobial properties of honey may be advantageous. Honey has also been shown to contain components that quench free radicals and act as anti-inflammatory agents (Henriques et al, 2006; Beretta et al, 2007; van den Berg et al, 2008), and, therefore, it may be able to interrupt the early damaging effects of radiation on cutaneous tissue.

Conclusion

Skin reactions and delayed post-operative wound healing is common in patients during radiotherapy and in those who have received treatment in the past (De Conno et al, 1991; Porock et al, 1999; MacBride et al, 2008). Although many different treatments have been suggested for the management of these wounds and the importance of selecting suitable dressings and topical treatments is recognised, there appears to be a lack of robust evidence to support any one treatment and variability remains within practice. Such wounds are often resistant to conventional therapy and pose a major problem as they may result in chronic ulceration and infection, heavily impacting on the patient's health and quality of life as well as draining economic resources. The lack of an assessment tool to evaluate irradiated skin reactions is an obstacle to the formulation of suitable clinical guidelines and helps to explain why none have yet been developed (Nystedt *et al*, 2005). Skin cleanliness, adequate hydration and the use of moist healing principles seem appropriate (Porock *et al* 1999; Wickline 2004; Nystedt *et al*, 2005). Several trials have evaluated various topical treatments and have raised the uncertainty of any treatment being effective in this area of care. This indicates that further research is warranted. Honey has not been subject to objective clinical evaluation in this field but the growing evidence in its use in chronic wound care merits its consideration in this demanding area. In Liverpool, honey is becoming increasingly popular in the management of ENT patients (Robson *et al*, 2007), and effective outcomes in managing radiation damaged skin are beginning to be reported (Robson and Cooper, 2009).

References

Bentzen SM, Overgaard J (1994) Seminars in radiation oncology. *Semin Radiation Oncol* 4(2): 53–4

Bentzen SM, Overgaard J (1994) Editorial. *Semin Radiation Oncol* 4(2): 53–4

Beretta G, Orloli M, Facino RM (2007) Antioxidant and radical scavenging activity of honey in endothelial cell cultures (EA.hy926). *Planta Medica* 73(11): 1182–9

Biswal BM, Zakaria A, Ahmad NM (2003) Topical application of honey in the management of radiation mucositis. A preliminary study. *Support Cancer Care* 11: 242–8

Borg M, Wilkinson D, Humeniuk V, Norman J (2001) Successful treatment of radiation-induced breast ulcer and hyperbaric oxygen. *The Breast* 10: 336–41

Cooper RA (2008) Using honey to inhibit wound pathogens. *Nurs Times* 104(3): 46–9

De Conno F, Ventafridda V, Saita L (1991) Skin problems in advanced and terminal cancer patients. *J Pain Symptom Management* 6: 247–56

Delaney GP, Jacob S, Featherstone C, Barton NB (2005) The role of radiotherapy in cancer treatment: estimating optimal utilisation from a review of evidence-based clinical guidelines. *Cancer* 104: 1129–37

Denham JW, Hauer-Jensen M (2002) The radiotherapeutic injury — a complex 'wound'. _Radiother Oncol_ **63**: 129–45

Dormand EL, Banwell PE, Goodacre TE (2005) Radiotherapy and wound healing. _Int Wound J_ **2**(2): 112–27

Henriques A, Jackson S, Cooper R, Burton N (2006) Free radical production and quenching in honeys with wound healing potential. _J Antimicrob Chemother_ **58**: 773–7

Holmes S (1988) _Radiotherapy_. Austin Cornish, London

Hom D B, Adams G, Koreis M, Maisel R (1999) Choosing the optimal wound dressing for irradiated soft tissue wounds. _Otolaryngol Head Neck Surg_ **121**: 591–8

Jemel A, Siegel R, Ward E, Taylor M, Xu J, Thun MJ (2007) Cancer statistics. _Cancer J Clin_ **57**: 43–66

MacBride S, Wells M, Hornsby C, Sharp L, Finnila K, Downie L (2008) A case study to evaluate a new soft silicone dressing, Mepilex Lite, for patients with radiation skin reactions. _Cancer Nurs_ **31**(1): E8–E14

Maddocks-Jennings, Wilkinson JM, Shillington D (2005) Novel approaches to radiotherapy-induced skin reactions: A literature review. _Complementary Therapies Clinical Practice_ **11**: 224–31

Mak S, Molassiotis A, Wan W, Lee I, Chan E (2000) The effects of hydrocolloid dressing and gentian violet on radiation-induced moist desquamation wound healing. _Cancer Nurs_ **23**(3): 220–9

Margolin SG, Breneman JC, Denman DL, LaChapelle P, Weckbach L, Aron BS (1990) Management of radiation-induced moist skin desquamation using hydrocolloid dressings. _Cancer Nurs_ **13**(2) : 71–80

McQuestion M (2006) Evidence-based skin care management. In: Radiation therapy. _Semin Oncol Nurs_ **22**(3): 163–73

Mendelsohn F, Divino CM, Kerstein ED (2002) Wound care after radiation therapy. _Adv Skin Wound Care_ **15**(5): 216–24

Moolenaar M, Poorter RL, van der Toorn PPG, _et al_ (2006) The effect of honey compared to conventional treatment on healing of radiotherapy-induced skin toxicity in breast cancer patients. _Acta Oncological_ **45**: 623–4

Motallebnejad M, Akram S, Moghadamnia A, _et al_ (2008) The effect of topical application of pure honey on radiation-induced mucositis: a randomized clinical trial. _J Comtemp Dent Pract_ **9**(3): 40–7

Nystedt KE, Hill JE, Mitchell AM, Goodwin F, Rowe LA, Wong LW, Kind A L (2005) The standardization of radiation skin care in British Columbia: a collaborative approach. _Oncol Nurs Forum_ **32**(6): 1199–1205

Olascoaga A, Vilar-Compte D, Poitevin-Chacon A, Contreras-Ruiz J (2008) Wound healing in radiated skin: pathophysiology and treatment options. _Int Wound J_ **5**(2): 246–57

Parkin DM, Bray F, Ferlay J, Pisani P (2005) Global Cancer Statistics, 2002. *Cancer J Clin* **55**: 74–108

Porock D (2002) Factors influencing the severity of radiation skin and oral mucosal reactions: development of a conceptual framework. *Eur J Cancer Care* **11**: 33–43

Porock D, Kristjanson L (1999) Skin reactions during radiotherapy for breast cancer: the use and impact of topical agents and dressings. *Eur J Cancer Care* **8**: 143–53

Porock D, Nikoletti S, Kristjanson L (1999) Management of radiation skin reactions: literature review and clinical applications. *Plast Surg Nurs* **19**: 4, 185–191

Rashad UK, Al-Gezawy SM, Azzazz AN, *et al* (2008) Honey as topical prophylaxis against radiotherapy-induced mucositis in head and neck cancer. *J Laryngol Otol* **19**: 1–6

Robson V, Cooper RA (in press for 2009) The use of *Leptospermum* honey in the management of wounds resulting from skin damage following radiotherapy in head and neck cancer patients. *Ostomy/Wound Management*

Robson V, Cooper RA, Ehsan ME (2007) The use of honey in wound management following ENT surgery. *Primary Intention* **15**(4): 176–80

Robson V, Martin L, Cooper RA (2005) The use of *Leptospermum* honey on chronic wounds in breast care. In: White R, Cooper R, Molan P, eds. *Honey: A modern wound management product*. Wounds UK, Aberdeen

Schimp V, Worley C, Brunello S, Lavenback C, Wolf J, Sun C, Bodurka D, Ramirez P (2004) Vacuum-assisted closure in the treatment of gynaecological oncology wound failures. *Gynaecol Oncol* **92**: 586–91

Stone HB, Coleman CN, Anscher MS, McBride WH (2003) Effects of radiation on normal tissue: consequences and mechanisms. *Lancet* Oncol **4**(9): 529–36

Thomas S (1992) *Current Practices in the Management of Fungating Lesions and Radiation Damaged Skin*. Surgical Materials Testing Laboratory, Bridgend, Mid-Glamorgan

van den Berg AJ, van den Worm E, van Ufford HC, Halkes SB, Hoekstra MJ, Beukelman CJ (2008) An *in vitro* examination of the antioxidant and anti-inflammatory properties of buckwheat honey. *J Wound Care* **17**(4): 172–4, 176–8

Wickline MM (2004) Prevention and treatment of acute radiation dermatitis: A literature review. *Oncol Nurs Forum* **31**(2): 237–47

CHAPTER 13

TOPICAL APPLICATION OF HONEY IN THE TREATMENT OF BURNS

Mutya Subrahmanyam and Stuart Enoch

Over the past couple of decades, management of burn wounds has improved with enhanced understanding of the pathophysiology of burns and wound healing mechanisms. Better appreciation of the working of the immune system and advances in diagnostic microbiology, combined with advances in tissue engineering and biological dressings has further helped to reduce the morbidity and mortality from burns. However, controlling infection, scarring and its associated problems poses a challenge for healthcare professionals (Subrahmanyam, 1996a). Likewise, the search for an optimal burn wound dressing that is cheap, practical, easily stored, that controls infection, minimises scarring and is easily available still remains elusive. Over the years, honey, that has many of the aforementioned properties, has been used to accelerate healing and to control infection in various types of wounds, including those due to burns. This chapter discusses the role of honey in the management of burns using an evidence-based approach.

Burn aetiology and depth

A burn can occur by a flame (flame/flash burns), a hot liquid (scalds) or a hot solid (contact burns). Other important causes for burns include chemicals (acids or alkalis), electricity or lightening strike, radiation, radioactivity and extreme cold (frost-bite). The classification of burns into four categories (superficial, superficial partial-thickness, deep partial-thickness and full-thickness) depends on the depth of tissue damage that has occurred and is directly linked to the temperature and duration of exposure to thermal extremes.

Burn severity and outcome

The severity of any burn injury is related to the size, depth and anatomical location of the burn. Studies evaluating the factors influencing outcome in burns have identified three risk factors for death:

1. Age above 60 years
2. Total body surface area (TBSA) involvement above 40%
3. Inhalation injury (Ryan, 1998).

It has been found in >40% TBSA burns that associated infection significantly increases overall mortality (Gupta *et al*, 1993).

However, unlike before, treatment outcome in burn patients is now measured not just by survival but also by health-related quality of life, including function and cosmesis. To this end, with improving survival outcomes (mortality about 5–6% in specialised centres) (Bloemsma *et al*, 2008), there is currently a shift of assessment of outcome from mortality to quality-of-life measures, such as the Short Form-36 (SF-36) and the Vineland Adaptive Behaviour Scales Survey Form (VABS-SF) (Pereira *et al*, 2004). The current focus in burn patients is the preservation of function, reconstruction and rehabilitation (Bloemsma *et al*, 2008) and, as such, the management of the skin in burns achieves enormous significance.

Pathophysiology of burns

Burn injury leads to complex pathophysiological alterations that exert a deleterious effect on various organ systems. Thermal injury of the skin, a form of oxidation injury, leads to an increase in xanthine oxidase activity that is accompanied by an increase in lipid peroxidation. The biological and metabolic alterations include:

* *Degradation of adenosine triphosphate:* a significant reduction in polyunsaturated fatty acids in the red cell membrane.
* *Elevation of activity of serum enzymes* (Nishikagi *et al*, 1980; Till *et al*, 1985; Kumar *et al*, 1995).

These changes are associated with the formation of the lipid peroxidation product malon dialdehyde. There is experimental evidence showing increased levels of lipid peroxide in rat serum and in burn patients after thermal injury (Nishikagi _et al_, 1980; Kumar _et al_, 1995). An elevated level of lipid peroxide in the serum in the early post-burn period reflects increased activity of free radicals. This can result in the generation of the lipid peroxidation products that are detected in burnt skin, serum and the lungs.

Infection in burn wounds

Infection and in some cases septicaemia is an important cause for mortality during the early phase in burn patients. Compromise of the immune function also contributes towards the development and persistence of infection. Prevention of infection is essential for optimal regeneration of the epithelial cells and/or lost dermis to occur. Wound swabs taken from the surface of the burn wound may identify superficial organisms but are not particularly useful in making the diagnosis of invasive infection. It has been identified that the surface cultures of burn wounds correlate poorly with the presence of invasive burn wound infection (Pruitt _et al_, 1991). Therefore, the microbiological examination of burn wound biopsy (a 3–4 mm punch biopsy) is the most reliable means of detecting invasive burn wound infection, as compared to surface cultures of the burn wound. _Pseudomonas_ and _Staphylococcus aureus_ are the most commonly isolated organisms in burn wounds (Subrahmanyam, 1991; Subrahmanyam _et al_, 2003b).

Choice of dressing for a burn wound

Epidermal regeneration in a burn wound is a complex process in which residual epithelial cells proliferate in a coordinated manner to form an intact epidermis. In superficial and partial-thickness burns, there are still a sufficient number of epithelial cells that survive within the hair follicles and sweat glands. A moist environment is the best suited for epithelialisation and wound healing (Winter, 1963). Thus, the key lies with dressings that are easy to apply, painless, simple to manage and widely available. To reduce bacterial growth under the burn surface and facilitate wound healing, various agents such as 1% silver sulfadiazine (Fox, 1975), 5% silver nitrate (Moyer _et al_, 1965), sulfamylon (Moncrief, 1974) and various synthetic and biological dressings with live cultured fibroblasts within the matrix have been used (Davies, 1984). However, none of these agents effectively control infection. Furthermore, the emergence of antibiotic-resistant pathogens makes it necessary to identify an alternative to counter these multi-drug resistant organisms.

Natural products are used in many parts of the world to enhance wound healing. A survey conducted by Hermans (1998) to review worldwide use of different treatment options for burns found that honey was used in 5.5% of instances in superficial burns, while 1% silver sulfadiazine was the preferred treatment for partial-thickness and deep burns. Since then, evidence has emerged to support the beneficial effects of honey in controlling infection and promoting wound healing in superficial and superficial partial thickness burns (Moore *et al*, 2001).

Honey as a medicinal wound healing product

The medicinal properties of honey have been known for centuries (*Chapter 1*). The Indian system of medicine, 'Ayurveda', describes honey as the 'nectar of life' and recommends its use in the treatment of various ailments such as diarrhoea and ulcers (*Chapter 1*). The many properties of honey, as described in this book, are widely recognised. It is nutritious, enhances the immune system and has been used for storing skin grafts (Subrahmanyam, 1993a; Postmes *et al*, 1993; Klein *et al*, 2000).

Mechanism of action of honey-based dressings

The components and features of honey that are relevant to wound healing are as follows: viscosity, water content, sugars (primarily glucose and fructose), antioxidants, a wide range of amino acids, vitamins and minerals, glucose oxidase, which produces hydrogen peroxide, and gluconic acid, which gives honey an acidic pH of 3.2 to 4.5. Hydrogen peroxide is produced only when the honey is diluted, as glucose oxidase is inhibited in undiluted honey — this provides most of the antibacterial activity of diluted honey (in undiluted honey the high osmolarity prevents bacterial growth [White *et al*, 1963]) and improves local nutrition because of the presence of laevulose and fructose (Molan, 2001). Numerous microbiological studies have shown the antibacterial effect of honey (Anand and Shanmugam, 1998; Efem *et al*, 1992; Subrahmanyam *et al*, 2001a; Molan, 1992; Cooper *et* _al_, 2002; Cooper _et al_, 1999; Molan, 2001) (_Chapter 3_). Wound swabs taken before and after honey treatment and conventional treatment have shown significantly reduced rates of infection in the former, indicating that honey minimises the bacterial count in wounds and promotes early granulation (Subrahmanyam, 1993b). Consequently, this results in early wound healing and decreased hospital stay; indirect evidence for the cost-effectiveness of treatment with honey.

Evidence for the use of honey in burn wounds

In 1933, Philips described the use of honey in burns and suggested it to be one of the best natural dressings. In 1937, Voigtlander used honey to treat scalds and highlighted the pain-relieving and soothing action honey provided. Studies in animal models have demonstrated that honey leads to quicker healing and reduced inflammation in superficial burns, as well as in certain deeper burns that are free from infection. In addition, rapid healing has also been observed in experimental wounds infected with _S. aureus_ (Postmes _et al_, 1997).

Isolated case reports have described superficial burn wounds healed with honey dressings that were refractory to conventional treatment (Efem, 1988). A retrospective study of 156 burn patients treated in a hospital over a five-year period (1988–1992) found that 13 patients treated with honey had a similar outcome to those treated with silver sulfadiazine (Adesunkamni and Olyelamy, 1994).

In a systematic review of trials of honey in burns and wounds, Moore _et al_ (2001) suggested that honey was superior to other treatments. It was reported in February of this year in the _New York Times_ that the Center for Disease Control in Atlanta, USA, had evaluated the evidence from various systematic trials using honey in burns and reported that it has antibacterial and anti-inflammatory activities that promote burn wound healing and soothe discomfort.

In a trial of 104 wounds (patients) comparing honey (52 wounds) and silver sulfadiazine (52 wounds), 91% of the wounds treated with honey were free of infection within seven days, compared to only 7% of wounds in the group treated with silver sulfadiazine. Likewise, healthy granulation tissue was observed earlier in patients treated with honey than those treated with silver sulfadiazine (mean 7.4 versus 13.4 days; $p < 0.05$). Of those dressed with honey, 87% of the wounds achieved complete healing within 15 days, compared with 10% of those treated with silver sulfadiazine. Furthermore, patients treated with honey dressings reported less pain, exudation and wound irritation (Subrahmanyam, 1991) (*Table 13.1*).

Table 13.1: Burn wounds treated with honey and silver sulfadiazine (Subrahmanyam, 1991)			
Treatment arm	Extent of burns in %	Free of infection within days	Wounds 100% healed after 15 days
Silver sulfadiazine (n=52)	5–40%	7%	10%
Honey (n=52)	5–40%	19%	87%

In another trial (Subrahmanyam, 1998) involving 50 patients comparing honey with silver sulfadiazine (25 patients in each arm), histological examination of biopsy samples from the wound margin as well as clinical observations of wound healing were made. By the seventh day, 84% of the wounds dressed with honey showed satisfactory epithelialisation compared with 72% of those dressed with silver sulfadiazine. By the twenty-first day, this increased to 100% in the honey-dressing group, compared with 84% in the silver sulfadiazine group. Histological evidence of reparative activity showed early subsidence of acute inflammatory changes in the honey-dressed wounds, whereas sustained inflammatory reaction was seen even on epithelialisation in the wounds treated with silver sulfadiazine. No skin grafting was required for the wounds treated with honey, but four wounds treated with silver sulfadiazine progressed to full-thickness and required skin grafting (Subrahmanyam, 2001b).

In the same study, healing was faster with honey, with a mean time of 15 days as against 17 days for the group treated with silver sulfadiazine. In the group treated with honey, 90% wounds were free of infection after one week, while infection persisted in the other group (Subrahmanyam *et al*, 2001b) (*Table 13.2*). The average hospital stay was 22 days in the group treated with honey, while it was 32 days in the group treated with silver sulfadiazine (Subrahmanyam *et al*, 2001b). Similar results have been reported in a study of burns in children (Bangroo *et al*, 2005).

Prospective randomised controlled clinical trials have also shown that treatment with honey leads to significantly more rapid healing of superficial and partial-thickness burns than that achieved with polyurethane film, amniotic membrane, and potato peels

Table 13.2: Healing rates with with honey and silver sulfadiazine (Subrahmanyam, 2001)			
Treatment	Cumulative number of % healed		
	Day 7	Day 14	Day 21
Honey (n=50)	8 (16%)	45 (90%)	50 (100%)
SSD (n=50)	4 (8%)	26 (52%	50 (100%)

(Subrahmanyam, 1993c; 1994; 1996b). However, in full-thickness burns, early tangential excision and skin grafting were found to be superior to honey dressings, although it needs to be acknowledged that honey may have a role in treating these wounds where facilities for early tangential excision and skin grafting are not available (Subrahmanyam, 1999). Thus, in superficial and partial-thickness burns, honey treatment has resulted in an effective control of infection that is better than that achieved with current standard treatment, silver sulfadiazine, and other modalities (Subrahmanyam, 1994; Subrahmanyam _et al_, 2001b; Bangroo _et al_, 2005).

The early application of honey may also mop up the free radicals (that result in increased lipid peroxidation) and thus have a role in reducing scarring and contractures; conclusive level 1 evidence is however lacking. This may also possibly explain the reduced depigmentation after treatment with honey compared to silver sulfadiazine and other treatment modalities (Subrahmanyam _et al_, 2003c).

Management of minor burns using honey

As part of first aid, once the patient is removed from the burning source, the burn should be cooled (or the toxin diluted) with luke-warm running water for at least 20 minutes. This period should be increased in those with chemical injury. Ice or very cold water should be avoided, as blood flow to the affected area will be reduced, and, consequently, result in hypothermia; infants and the elderly are particularly susceptible. Simple analgesia or opiates should be used. In the initial stages, covering the burn and cooling with water will also provide some pain relief.

Removal of burn debris with mild soap and water, sterile saline or a topical antiseptic solution should be performed, prior to application of a honey-based dressing. The dead skin of open blisters should be removed and large or friable blisters should also be de-roofed. Small blisters may be left intact. Depending on the area, 15–30 ml of honey sterilised by gamma irradiation can be applied directly onto the burn wound or soaked in gauze before application. Occlusive or absorbent secondary dressings may be necessary to prevent honey from oozing out. A clean wound bed before the application of the honey-based dressing is preferable, but not essential. Antibiotics are not routinely prescribed in minor burns. The tetanus status of the patient should be checked.

Repeated review of the burn wound and multiple dressing changes are usually unnecessary. A change of dressings and wound review after 48 hours is sufficient in most instances. Further changes will be guided by the rate of healing (generally 2–3 day intervals). More frequent dressing changes may be required if there is a high volume of exudate (Subrahmanyam, 2007) or evidence of infection.

Conclusion

In summary, based on current scientific evidence, there is a proven role for the use of dressings based on honey derivatives in superficial and superficial partial-thickness burns. They minimise the risk of infection, reduce pain during dressing changes, promote granulation tissue formation and epithelialisation, and provide a moist environment that is conducive to rapid wound healing. The role of honey dressings in wounds that are overtly infected, or those with excessive amounts of slough and necrotic tissue in the wound bed is not yet conclusively established. Furthermore, there is currently insufficient evidence to support the routine use of honey in the treatment of deep partial-thickness and full-thickness burns.

References

Adesunkamni K, Olyelamy OA (1994) The pattern and outcome of burn injuries in West Guilds Hospital, Ilesha, Nigeria: A review of 156 cases. *J Trop Med Hyg* 97: 108–12

Anand A, Shanmugam J (1998) Antistaphylococcal properties of natural honey. *Biomedicine* 18: 15–8

Bangroo AK, Khatri R, Chauhan S (2005) Honey dressing in paediatric burns. *J Indian Assoc Paediatr Surgeons* 10: 172–5

Bloemsma GC, Dokter J, Boxma H, Oen IM (2008) Mortality and causes of death in a burn centre. _Burns_ June 5 [Epub ahead of print]

Cooper RA, Hakas, Molan PC (2002) The efficacy of honey in inhibiting strains of _Pseudomonas aureginosa_ from infected burns. _J Burn Care Rehabil_ 23: 366–70

Cooper RA, Molan PC, Harding KG (1999) Antibacterial activity of honey against strains of _Staphylococcus aureus_ from infected wounds. _J ER Soc Med_ 9: 283–5

Davies JWL (1984) Synthetic materials fore covering burn wounds. Progress towards perfection 1. short term materials. _Burns_ 10: 94–103

Efem SE (1988) Clinical observations on the wound healing properties of honey. _Br J Surg_ 75: 679–81

Efem SE, Udoh KT, Iwara CL (1992) The antimicrobial spectrum of honey and its clinical significance. _Infection_ 20: 227–9

Fox CL Jr (1975) Silver sulphadiazine for control of burn wound infection. _Int Surg_ 60: 275–7

Gupta M, Gupta OK, Yaduvanshi RK, _et al_ (1993) Burn epidemiology. The pink city scene. _Burns_ 19: 47–51

Hermans MHE (1998) Results of a survey on the use of different treatment options for partial and full thickness burns. _Burns_ 24: 539–51

Klein C, Sato T, Meguid MM, Miyata G (2000) From food to nutritional support to specific nutraceuticals: a journey across time in the treatment of disease. _J Gastroenterol_ 35(12): 1–6

Kumar M, Seth RK, Sekhon MS, Bhargava JS (1995) Serum lipid peroxide and other enzyme levels of patients suffering from thermal injury. _Burns_ 21: 96–7

Molan PC (1992) The antibacterial effect of honey. 1. The nature of antibacterial activity. _Bee World_ 73: 5–28

Molan PC (2001) Potential of honey in the treatment of wounds and burns. _Am J Clin Dermatol_ 2: 13–19

Moncrief JA (1974) Topical antibacterial therapy for burn wound. _Clin Plastic Surg_ 1: 563–76

Moore OA, Smith LA, Campbell D, _et al_ (2001) Systematic review of the use of honey as a wound dressing. _BMC Complement Altern Med_ 1: 28

Moyer CA, Brentano L, Gravens DL, Margraf NW, Manafo WW (1965) Treatment of large human burns with 5% silver nitrate solution. _Arch Surg_ 90: 812–67

Nishikagi K, Hagihara M, Hiramatsu M, Tawy Y, Yagi K (1980) Effect of thermal injury on lipid peroxide levels of rat. _Biochem Med_ 24: 185–9

Pereira C, Murphy K, Herndon D (2004) Outcome measures in burn care: Is mortality dead? _Burns_ 30: 761–71

Philips CEE (1933) Honey for burns. _Gleanings in Bee Culture_ 61: 284

Postmes T, van den Bogaard AE, Hazen M (1993) Honey for wounds, ulcers, and skin graft preservation. _Lancet_ 341(8847): 756–7

Postmes T, Bosch MMC, Butrireux R, _et al_ (1997) Speeding up the healing of burns with honey. An experimental study with histological assessment of wound biopsies. In: Mzrahi, Lensky, eds. *Bee Products*. Plenum Press, New York: 57–63

Pruitt BA Jr, Goodwin GW Jr, Pruitt SJ (1991) In: Sabisten BG Jr, ed. *Text Book of Surgery*. 14th edn. WB Saunders, Philadelphia: 199

Ryan CM, Schoenfeld DA, Thorpe WP, Sheridan RL, Cassem EH, Tompkins RG (1998) Objective estimates of the probability of death from burn injuries. *N Engl J Med* **338**(6): 362–6

Subrahmanyam M (1991) Topical application of honey in treatment of burns. *Br J Surg* **78**: 497–8

Subrahmanyam M (1993a) Storage of skin grafts in honey. *Lancet* **341**(8836): 63–4

Subrahmanyam M (1993b) Honey as a surgical dressing for burns and ulcers. *Indian J Surg* **55**: 468–73

Subrahmanyam M (1993c) Honey-impregnated gauze versus polyurethane film (Opsite®) in the treatment of burns. *Br J Plast Surg* **46**: 322–3

Subrahmanyam M (1994) Honey-impregnated gauze versus amniotic membrane in the treatment of burns. *Burns* **20**: 331–3

Subrahmanyam M (1996a) Honey dressings for burns: An appraisal. *Ann Burns Fire Disasters* **9**: 33–5

Subrahmanyam M (1996b) Honey dressing versus boiled potato peel in the treatment of burns: a prospective randomized study. *Burns* **22**: 491–3

Subrahmanyam M (1998) A prospective randomized clinical and histological study of superficial burn wound healing with honey and silver sulphadiazine. *Burns* **24**: 157–61

Subrahmanyam M (1999) Early tangential excision and skin grafting of moderate burns is superior to honey dressings for burns. *Burns* **25**: 729–31

Subrahmanyam M (2007) Topical application of honey in treatment of burns — an overview. *Ann Burns Fire Disasters* **20**: 137–9

Subrahmanyam M, Archan M, Pawar SG (2001a) Antibacterial activity of honey on bacteria isolated from wounds. *Ann Burns Fire Disasters* **14**: 22–4

Subrahmanyam M, Shahapure AG, Nagne NS, *et al* (2001b) Effects of topical application of honey on burn wound healing. *Ann Burns Fire Disasters* **14**: 143–5

Subrahmanyam M, Hemmady AR, Pawar SG (2003a) The sensitivity of honey of multidrug-resistant *Pseudomonas aeruginosa* from infected burns. *Ann Burns Fire Disasters* **26**: 135–7

Subrahmanyam M, Hemmady AR, Pawar SG (2003b) Multidrug-resistant *Staphylococcus aureus* isolated from infected burns sensitive to honey. *Ann Burns Fire Disasters* **16**: 192–3

Subrahmanyam M, Shahapure AG, Nagne NS, *et al* (2003c) Free radical control – the main mechanism of action of honey in burns. *Ann Burns Fire Disasters* **14**: 135–7

Till GO, Hathreall JR, Tourtellette WW, Lutz BA, Ward PA (1985) Lipid peroxidation and acute lung injury after thermal trauma to the skin. *Am J Pathol* **119**: 376–84

Voigtlander N (1937) Honey for burns and scalds. _Bee World_ **18**: 128

Wadhan HAL (1998) Causes of antimicrobial activity of honey. _Infection_ **126**: 26–31

White JW Jr, Subers M, Schepartz AL (1963) The identification of 'inhibine', the antibacterial factor in honey as hydrogen peroxide and its origin in a honey glucose oxidase system. _Biochem Biophys Acta_ **73**: 57–70

Winter GD (1963) A note on wound healing under dressings with special reference to perforated dressings. _J Invest Dermatol_ **45**: 299

CHAPTER 14

IMMUNOMODULATORY COMPONENTS OF HONEY

Amanda Tonks

The healing properties of honey have been described for many centuries, and while there is an increasing body of scientific literature to support the use of honey as a wound healing agent, many aspects remain less understood. The scientific basis for the activities ascribed to honey are not well studied, with the components responsible for activity and their mechanisms of action yet to be fully elucidated. To date, a number of key properties of honey have been described and supported in the scientific literature, including the antimicrobial and immune stimulatory activities of honey. In these areas, attempts have been made to identify the components responsible for activity and determine the mode of action.

Honey is a complex mixture which is mainly composed of a number of key sugars, including fructose, glucose, maltose and sucrose, and small amounts of proteins, amino acids and lipids are present as well as low levels of vitamins and minerals. Many studies have identified contaminants in honey, ranging from pollen and royal jelly to bacterial spores or antibiotics and chemicals used to prevent disease in the hive (Martel *et al*, 2006; Tananaki *et al*, 2006). Generally, honey contains little bacterial contamination, largely due to the ability of bee colonies to eliminate pathogenic and non-pathogenic microbes. In addition, the physico-chemical properties of honey itself and the excellent chemical filtering performed by bees results in little chemical contamination of honey. The presence of chemical and microbial contaminants varies, as discussed in *Chapter 5*. However, when investigating the components present in honey responsible for the biological activity, it is important that all possibilities are considered.

Advanced glycation end-products present in honey

The antibacterial activity of honey is well characterised and has been reviewed in *Chapter 3*. Manuka honey has long been associated with a non-peroxide antibacterial activity, which has been assessed and quoted as unique manuka factor (UMF) (Allen *et al*, 1991). The UMF has recently been reported to be identified following isolation of a fraction of manuka honey which gives rise to the non-peroxide antibacterial activity of honey (Adams *et al*, 2008). The active component was suggested to be methylglyoxal (MG), with levels detected in honey correlating to UMF or non-peroxide antibacterial activity (Mavric *et al*, 2008). MG is a natural product which is synthesised by green photosynthesising plants. The production of this substance and its metabolites in plants are affected by environmental conditions such as salinity, drought and cold stresses (Adams *et al*, 2008), as well as by key detoxification/regulatory glyoxylase enzyme pathways (Yadav *et al*, 2008). The levels of MG in plants can be significantly affected (2–3-fold enhancement) by the conditions under which plants are grown (Yadav *et al*, 2005). The levels of MG in manuka honey are thought to be higher than in other honeys due to the marginal conditions in which the manuka plants (*Leptospermum scoparium*) grow (Adams *et al*, 2008). MG and other similar reactive 1, 2-dicarbonyl compounds are also byproducts of various metabolic pathways present in mammals, and are produced from carbohydrates in food and beverages during degradation and cooking processes. These reactions confer desirable taste and colour characteristics (Adams *et al*, 2008), but within biological systems these products (MG and 1, 2-dicarbonyl compounds) can have adverse effects. MG and similar products are highly reactive and have the ability to bind to important biological molecules such as proteins, lipids and DNA forming advanced glycation end-products (AGE). This affects not only the structure of these molecules, but also their function and metabolism (Price and Knight, 2007). AGE molecules have been linked to the pathogenesis of a number of diseases including atherosclerosis and diabetic vascular complications (Goh and Cooper, 2008). The addition of sugar molecules to protein, or glycation, occurs where there are raised levels of certain (reducing) sugars and reactive oxygen species (ROS), e.g. oxygen free radicals. This gives rise to proteins with altered structures and functions. These can interact with the receptors on many cell surfaces to elicit inflammatory responses and vascular damage. This is of particular clinical significance in diabetes (Nogueira-Machado and Chaves, 2008). AGE molecules can also accumulate intracellularly and are likely to play an important role in altering the function of intracellular proteins and activating intracellular signalling pathways (Giardino *et al*, 1994). AGE molecules bind to and activate a specific receptor for advanced glycation end-products (RAGE) (Ramasamy *et al*, 2008). This receptor interacts with a wide variety of ligands of this class and belongs to the immunoglobulin superfamily of receptors. Engagement of the receptor in monocytes, macrophages and endothelial cells activates proinflammatory, intracellular signalling pathways, culminating in activation of NF-kappaB (NF-kB) and upregulation of ICAM-1, VCAM-1, vascular endothelial growth factor (VEGF), interleukin-6 (IL-6) and tumour necrosis factor-alpha (TNF-α) expression/production (Goh and Cooper, 2008). This ultimately mediates enhanced cellular migration and upregulation of proinflammatory and prothrombotic molecular pathways (Ramasamy *et al*, 2008), contributing to vascular damage. Much of the biomedical research data available to date relating to MG and AGE has focused on the damaging effects of these molecules, however, studies have emerged (Kang *et al*, 1996; Milanesa *et al*, 2000) which indicate that MG may have anti-tumorgenic effects. Specifically, MG is believed to stimulate cells of the immune system to attack tumour cells (Bhattacharyya *et al*, 2008).

While the role of MG and consequently AGE molecules in vascular pathologies is well established, there is little evidence to suggest that honey or the MG component has detrimental effects on host cells and consequently, wound healing processes, when applied as an external dressing agent. While free radicals are liberated at the wound site by cells present and by honey itself; honey has been shown to have antioxidant properties (Henriques *et al*, 2006; see *Chapter 2*) which would help to reduce formation of AGE products locally. Indeed, it is possible that MG may aid wound healing processes by stimulating immune cells directly to produce inflammatory mediators, which may have a role in wound healing processes.

In addition to naturally occurring products, a number of contaminants isolated from honey have antibacterial properties. These include antibiotics used to treat hives against foul brood, such as tetracycline, which have been directly detected in honey samples (Martel *et al*, 2006). Some of the most potent antimicrobial compounds known to man are derived from bacterial and fungal species, and all the antibiotics we have relied so heavily upon in recent times are derived from, or modelled on, naturally occurring microbial products.

Many research groups have described contamination of honey with a wide variety of bacterial species, including spore forming potentially clinically important species such as _Clostridium botulinum_ (Snowdon and Cliver, 1996; Nevas _et al_, 2005). A recent study isolated over two thousand bacterial strains from only eight different honey samples. The isolated microbes were found to inhibit the growth of bacterial strains including _Listeria monocytogenes_ and _Bacillus_ sp., as well as exhibiting antifungal activity (Lee _et al_, 2008).

Immune stimulatory components present in honey and their potential role in wound healing

Normal wound healing is a complex and dynamic process in which damaged tissue is removed and gradually replaced by restorative tissue during an overlapping series of events that include inflammation, tissue formation and tissue remodelling (Moseley _et al_, 2004; Falanga, 2005; Eming _et al_, 2007; Werner _et al_, 2007). The process involves interactions between extracellular matrix components (ECM), soluble mediators including cytokines, resident and infiltrating inflammatory cells and dermal and epidermal cell populations (Eming _et al_, 2007; Gallucci _et al_, 2004). To date, the role of honey in wound healing has mostly been studied in relation to its ability to stimulate aspects of the inflammatory response.

The initial inflammatory phase of healing has an essential role in clearing the wound site of infectious agents and debris; this is facilitated by the activities of innate immune cells, such as neutrophils and macrophages. These white blood cells migrate to the wound site in response to tissue damage and utilising their phagocytic abilities, clear the area of bacteria and debris, including dead and damaged cells, thus providing a cleared canvas for tissue repair (Leibovich and Ross 1975; DiPietro, 1995; Dovi _et al_, 2003; Duffield _et al_, 2005; Martin and Leibovich 2005). The importance of these cells in wound healing has been investigated and, while a reduction in the number of neutrophils present at the wound site expedites healing (Dovi _et al_, 2003), the depletion of macrophages is associated with poor debridement of the wound site and delayed repair (Leibovich and Ross, 1975; Duffield _et al_, 2005). Explanations have been put forward for these phenomena, specifically the fact that neutrophils constitute much of the debris present at the wound site: it is thought that reduction in their numbers may prove beneficial to healing so long as infectious agents and wound debris can be cleared effectively by resident and infiltrating macrophages (see *Chapter 2*). Regarding the essential role of macrophages in wound healing, in addition to their phagocytic role, macrophages release various growth factors and cytokines which are important in perpetuating the healing process, and thus encourage healing (Gillitzer and Goebeler, 2001).

A number of *in vivo* studies (Gaspari, 2000; LaDuca and Gaspari, 2001) indicate that production of key mediators, such as IL-6 and TNF-α by macrophages, and other cells at the wound site are essential in the healing process. Mice in which the gene for IL-6 has been knocked out exhibit delayed cutaneous healing compared to wildtype controls, with minimal migration and decreased inflammation and granulation at the wound site. This culminated in a three-fold increase in healing time. This delay could be rapidly reversed by treatment with recombinant murine IL-6 (Gallucci *et al*, 2000).

The production of mediators like IL-6 and TNF-α is part of the normal inflammatory response which facilitates infiltration of white blood cells into the wound site to aid clearance of microbes and cellular debris. The production of these mediators can be induced by interactions of key receptors on the surface of cells with components of bacterial, viral or fungal species, or by interactions with endogenous components including cell and extracellular matrix breakdown products such as hyaluronan which are generated in tissue injury (Termeer *et al*, 2002). A wide spectrum of receptors have been identified which are able to recognise these ligands, these receptors are sometimes referred to as pattern recognition receptors (PRRs), the most well characterised group of receptors are the Toll-like receptors (TLRs).

Toll-like receptors are a family of cellular membrane receptors found in a wide range of cell types, with highest distribution being on the membranes of inflammatory cells. To date, more than ten TLRs have been identified in mammalian species (Akira, 2006). The signalling pathways initiated by receptor interactions are fairly well characterised, as are the ligands required for activation of the different TLRs. These receptors allow recognition of a wide variety of conserved structures present across a plethora of microbial species of bacteria, viruses and fungi. These structures are sometimes referred to as pathogen or microbe-associated molecular patterns (PAMPs or MAMPs), since they recognise conserved structures on microbes, such as lipopolysaccharide (LPS), an outer membrane component of Gram-negative bacteria, or specific carbohydrate patterns found on the surface of fungi. These receptors also recognise a variety of host endogenous ligands, including cellular breakdown products which facilitate the removal of cell debris and aid tissue repair and homeostasis (Zhang and Schluesener, 2006).

Our group and others have previously shown that a variety of bee products including honey, propolis and royal jelly can stimulate production of inflammatory cytokines in various inflammatory cells. We have demonstrated that honey types (including manuka) can stimulate human peripheral blood monocytes (PBMCs) to produce inflammatory cytokines (e.g. TNF-α, IL-6, ILK-1) (Tonks _et al_, 2003; Tonks _et al_, 2007). Since previous studies indicate that honey can contain microbes, it is not unreasonable to suggest that the effects observed are largely due to the presence of microbes or some of their cellular components, indeed, the presence of LPS in honey has been determined in a number of studies (Tonks _et al_, 2003; Tonks _et al_, 2007; Timm _et al_, 2008). The results obtained in a study by Timm _et al_ (2008) examining a limited number of honey samples, concluded that activity was due to the presence of LPS in honey. This is in direct contrast to work published by our group which demonstrated that the observed effects of honey on cytokine production in myeloid cells are not a consequence of bacterial contamination of honey, nor the presence of LPS, but specifically associated with a 5.8 kDa moiety isolated from manuka honey (Tonks _et al_, 2007). The discrepancy in findings could be due to the large difference in numbers of bacteria which can be found in different samples of honey (see _Chapter 5_). Specifically, with regard to the data associated with manuka honey, we have surveyed a large number of manuka honey batches of known provenance to determine immune stimulatory activity. The samples were subjected to microbial analysis and quantitation of LPS using the limulus amoebocyte lysate (LAL) assay. All batches were found to be negative for vegetative bacterial growth, but around a third of samples were found to contain low levels of bacterial spores, and low levels of LPS were measured in all samples. Further, no correlation was found between the presence of bacterial spores or LPS levels and induction of the production of cytokines (Tonks _et al_, 2007), and levels of LPS detected were insufficient to stimulate production of the levels of cytokine observed in the study. The role of LPS in specific biological activities is generally confirmed in a number of ways, while the LAL assay is an excellent and sensitive method for measuring most species of LPS, some bacterial LPS is not easily detected by this method, and, commonly, additional assessments are undertaken to determine whether LPS is associated with an observed biological effect. These include the heating of components, since LPS molecules are not affected by heating, or, alternatively, the use of specific neutralising agents such as polymyxin B or LPS specific antibodies which bind to the active groups of LPS molecules and prevent their biological activity. The data from our study shows that the component present in honey which stimulates inflammatory cytokine synthesis is not inhibited by the presence of polymyxin and is significantly affected by heating, both indicating that the activity observed is likely to be independent of LPS.

Fractionation of the honey resulted in identification of an active fraction and subsequently purification of a specific 5.8 kDa component which stimulated induction of cytokines. Since cytokine production in inflammatory cells can be induced via activation of specific pattern recognition receptors, the role of these receptors in this mechanism were investigated. The 5.8 kDa component was found to stimulate cytokine production via the TLR4 receptor. This was confirmed in bone marrow-derived macrophages from mice in which the gene for TLR4 had been knocked out and in human peripheral blood monocytes utilising TLR4 blocking antibodies (Tonks *et al*, 2007). The chemical identity of the component is currently under investigation.

In a similar study, Simuth *et al* (2004) focused on royal jelly contaminants present in honey. Initial studies by these authors identified two key royal jelly proteins present in honey, namely apalbumin 1 and 2 (Apa 1 and 2). These proteins were found to stimulate mouse macrophages to release TNF-α (Simuth *et al*, 2004). Further, when the protein was produced in recombinant form of various lengths the activity was retained, indicating a link with activity. The importance of the protein moiety in eliciting this activity was further supported by evidence that while native honey can stimulate murine macrophages to produce TNF-α, deproteinated honey did not stimulate TNF-α release in these cells. Additionally, partial trypsin digestion of the recombinant protein resulted in alterations in activity, indicating the importance of key structural signatures (Majtan 2006). The recombinant protein was produced in *E.coli* bacteria, and during the purification process it is not unreasonable to consider that the protein preparation may have been contaminated with the bacterial cell wall component LPS. There is no indication of whether LPS levels were assessed in the protein preparations, and are therefore discrete from the activity of any LPS present in honey. However, the effect of trypsin digestion and differences seen in different truncated proteins indicate that the effects are associated with the protein, and not with LPS contamination.

Conclusion

While work to date has identified a number of discreet components with the potential to affect aspects of the wound healing process, whether that be associated with inhibition of microbial growth or initiation of the inflammatory phase of healing, there are likely to be many more components present which stimulate host cells to respond in various ways. In the future, the identification of active components may facilitate the production of fortified honey wound dressings with enhanced efficacy, or may lead to the production of honey-derived, chemically synthesised immune modulators or antimicrobials for multiple applications. Our group and others are working toward identifying key components and their mechanisms of action, which will facilitate advancements in this area. It is essential to assess the importance of crosstalk between inflammatory cells and fibroblasts in the process and determine key pathways involved in honey-mediated healing. By doing so, we may unlock the key to the full wound healing potential of honey.

References

Adams GJ, Boult GH, Deadman BJ, Farr JM, Grainger MN, Manley-Harris M, Snow MJ (2008) Isolation by HPLC and characterisation of the bioactive fraction of New Zealand manuka (*Leptospermum scoparium*) honey. *Carbohydr Res* 343(4): 651–9

Akira S (2006) TLR signalling. *Curr Top Microbiol Immunol* 311: 1–16

Allen KL, Molan PC, Reid GM (1991) A survey of the antibacterial activity of some New Zealand honeys. *J Pharm Pharmacol* 43(12): 817–22

Bhattacharyya N, Pal A, Patra S, Halder AK, Roy S, Ray M (2008) Activation of macrophages and lymphocytes by methylglyoxal against tumour cells in the host. *Int Immunopharmacol* July 7. E-pub ahead of print

Dimitrova B, Gevrenova R, Anklam E (2007) Analysis of phenolic acids in honeys of different floral origin by solid-phase extraction and high-performance liquid chromatography. *Phytochem Anal* 18(1): 24–32

DiPietro LA (1995) Wound healing: the role of the macrophage and other immune cells. *Shock* 4(4): 233–40

Dovi JV, He LK, DiPietro LA (2003) Accelerated wound closure in neutrophil-depleted mice. *J Leukoc Biol* 73(4): 448–55

Duffield JS, Forbes SJ, Constandinou CM, Clay S, Partolina M, Vuthoori S, Wu S, Lang R, Iredale JP (2005) Selective depletion of macrophages reveals distinct, opposing roles during liver injury and repair. *J Clin Invest* 115(1): 56–65

Eming SA, Krieg T, Davidson JM (2007) Inflammation in wound repair: molecular and cellular mechanisms. *J Invest Dermatol* **127**(3): 514–25.

Falanga V (2005) Wound healing and its impairment in the diabetic foot. *Lancet* **366**(9498): 1736–43

Gallucci RM, Simeonova PP, Matheson JM, Kommineni C, Guriel JL, Sugawara T, Luster MI (2000) Impaired cutaneous wound healing in interleukin-6-deficient and immunosuppressed mice. *FASEB J* **14**(15): 2525–31

Gallucci RM, Sloan DK, Heck JM, Murray AR, O'Dell SJ (2004) Interleukin 6 indirectly induces keratinocyte migration. *J Invest Dermatol* **122**(3): 764–72

Giardino I, Edelstein D, Brownlee M (1994) Nonenzymatic glycosylation *in vitro* and in bovine endothelial cells alters basic fibroblast growth factor activity. A model for intracellular glycosylation in diabetes. *J Clin Invest* **94**: 110–17

Gillitzer R, Goebeler M (2001) Chemokines in cutaneous wound healing. *J Leukoc Biol* **69**(4): 513–21

Goh SY, Cooper ME (2008) The role of advanced glycation end products in progression and complications of diabetes. *J Clin Endocrinol Metab* **93**(4): 1143–52

Henriques A, Jackson S, Cooper RA, Burton N (2006) Free radical production and quenching in honeys with wound healing properties. *J Antimicrob Chemother* **58**(4): 773–7

Kang Y, Edwards LG, Thornalley PJ (1996) Effect of methylglyoxal on human leukaemia 60 cell growth: modification of DNA G1 growth arrest and induction of apoptosis. *Leuk Res* **20**(5): 397–405

Lee H, Churey JJ, Worobo RW (2008) Antimicrobial activity of bacterial isolates from different floral sources of honey. *Int J Food Microbiol* **126**(1–2): 240–4

Leibovich SJ, Ross R (1975) The role of the macrophage in wound repair. A study with hydrocortisone and antimacrophage serum. *Am J Pathol* **78**(1): 71–100

Majtan J, Kovacova E, Bilikova K, Simuth J (2006) The immunostimulatory effect of the recombinant apalbumin 1- major honeybee royal jelly protein on TNF-alpha release. *Int Immunopharmacol* **6**(2): 269–78

Martel AC, Zeggane S, Drajnudel P, Faucon JP, Aubert M (2006) Tetracycline residues in honey after hive treatment. *Food Addit Contam* **23**(3): 265–73

Martin P, Leibovich SJ (2005) Inflammatory cells during wound repair: the good, the bad and the ugly. *Trends Cell Biol* **15**(11): 599–607

Mavric E, Wittmann S, Barth G, Henle T (2008) Identification and quantification of methylglyoxal as the dominant antibacterial constituent of manuka (*Leptospermum scoparium*) honeys from New Zealand. *Mol Nutr Food Res* **52**(4): 483–9

Milanesa DM, Choudhury MS, Mallouh C, Tazaki H, Konno S (2000) Methylglyoxal-induced apoptosis in human prostate carcinoma: potential modality for prostate cancer treatment. *Eur Urol* **37**(6): 728–34

Moseley R, Stewart JE, Stephens P, Waddington RJ, Thomas DW (2004) Extracellular matrix metabolites as potential biomarkers of disease activity in wound fluid:

lessons learned from other inflammatory diseases? *Br J Dermatol* **150**(3): 401–13

Nevas M, Lindstrom M, Hautamaki K, Puoskari S, Korkeala H (2005) Prevalence and diversity of *Clostridium botulinum* types A, B, E and F in honey produced in the Nordic countries. *Int J Food Microbiol* **105**(2): 145–51

Nogueira-Machado JA, Chaves MM (2008) From hyperglycemia to AGE-RAGE interaction on the cell surface: a dangerous metabolic route for diabetic patients. *Expert Opin Ther Targets* **12**(7): 871–82

Price CL, Knight SC (2007) Advanced glycation: a novel outlook on atherosclerosis. *Curr Pharm Des* **13**(36): 3681–7

Ramasamy R, Yan SF, Herold K, Clynes R, Schmidt AM (2008) Receptor for advanced glycation end products, fundamental roles in inflammatory response. *Ann N Y Acad Sci* **1126**: 7–13

Simuth J, Bilikova K, Kovacova E, Kuzmova Z, Schroder W (2004) Immunological approach to detection of adulteration in honey: physiologically active royal jelly protein stimulating TNF-alpha release is a regular component of honey. *J Agric Food Chem* **52**(8): 2154–8

Snowdon JA, Cliver DO (1996) Microorganisms in honey. *Int J Food Microbiol* **31**(1–3): 1–26

Tananaki C, Thrasyvoulou A, Karazafiris E, Zotou A (2006) Contamination of honey by chemicals applied to protect honeybee combs from wax-moth (*Galleria mellonela L.*). *Food Addit Contam* **23**(2): 159–63

Termeer C, Benedix F, Sleeman J, Fieber C, Voith U, Ahrens T, *et al* (2002) Oligosaccharides of Hyaluronan activate dendritic cells via toll-like receptor 4. *J Exp Med* **195**(1): 99–111

Timm M, Bartelt S, Hansen EW (2008) Immunomodulatory effects of honey cannot be distinguished from endotoxin. *Cytokine* **42**(1): 113–20

Tonks AJ, Cooper RA, Jones KP, Blair S, Parton J, Tonks A (2003) Honey stimulates inflammatory cytokine production from monocytes. *Cytokine* **21**(5): 242–7

Tonks AJ, Dudley E, Porter NG, Parton J, Brazier J, Smith EL, Tonks A (2007) A 5.8-kDa component of manuka honey stimulates immune cells via TLR4. *J Leukoc Biol* **82**(5): 1147–55

Wahdan HA (1998) Causes of the antimicrobial activity of honey. *Infection* **26**(1): 26–31

Werner S, Krieg T, Smola H (2007) Keratinocyte-fibroblast interactions in wound healing. *J Invest Dermatol* **127**(5): 998–1008

Yadav SK, Singla-Pareek SL, Sopory SK (2008) An overview on the role of methylglyoxal and glyoxalases in plants. *Drug Metabol Drug Interact* **23**(1–2): 51–68

Yadav SK, Singla-Pareek SL, Ray M, Reddy MK, Sopory SK (2005) Methylglyoxal levels in plants under salinity stress are dependent on glyoxalase I and glutathione. *Biochem Biophys Res Commun* **337**(1): 61–7

Zhang Z, Schluesener HJ (2006) Mammalian toll-like receptors: from endogenous ligands to tissue regeneration. *Cell Mol Life Sci* **63**(24): 2901–7

INDEX